ABOUT TH

Dr Guang Xu graduated from ~~~~~~~~
Traditional Chinese Medicir~~~~~~~~
Subsequently, she worked in the Comparative Department
of Traditional Chinese and Modern Western Medicine at
The Shanghai Seamen's Hospital for six years before she
came to work in London.

The Seamen's Hospital is a well-equipped hospital for
seamen and travellers from all over the world, and is well
known as one of the training hospitals for foreign TCM
students. Having worked in such an international hospital,
Dr Xu was able to practise the best of the traditional remedies as well as those of the new. She prides herself on
having gained her clinical experience in a combative sense
– that is, not just accepting held truths but testing them to
the limit. This gave her a deeper insight into all aspects of
her profession.

In 1989, the Chinese Government offered Dr Xu the
chance to work in London, to help spread knowledge of
traditional medicine within a modern context. Since then,
she has worked in a number of Chinese medical centres, as
well as teaching at the School of Chinese Herbal Medicine.
Since 1992, she has worked closely with Dr David
Atherton, consultant dermatologist at Great Ormond Street
Hospital for Children, exchanging knowledge, especially
about the treatment of skin conditions.

She currently runs a busy clinic in Chiswick, West
London and is regarded as one of the best TCM practitioners in the UK.

CHINESE HERBAL MEDICINE

A practical guide to the healing power of herbs

Dr Guang Xu

To
Lauren & Mrs Cox

Love from

[signature]

V

VERMILION
LONDON

1 3 5 7 9 10 8 6 4 2

First published in the United Kingdom in 1996 by Vermilion
an imprint of Ebury Press
Random House
20 Vauxhall Bridge Road
London SW1V 2SA

Random House Australia (Pty) Limited
20 Alfred Street, Milsons Point, Sydney,
New South Wales 2061, Australia

Random House New Zealand Limited
18 Poland Road, Glenfield,
Auckland 10, New Zealand
Random House South Africa (Pty) Limited
PO Box 337, Bergvlei, South Africa

Random House UK Limited Reg. No. 954009

A CIP catalogue record for this book is available from the British Library.

ISBN: 0 09 180944 4

Illustrations: Stephen Dew

Designed and typeset from author's disk by Bob Vickers
Printed and bound in Great Britain by
Mackays of Chatham PLC , Chatham, Kent

Papers used by Ebury Press are natural recyclable products made from wood
grown in sustainable forests.

Contents

Preface

My mother used to be a "medicine bottle" (a Chinese expression
for people who always take lots of medicine) when I was a child;
it was really upsetting to see my mother suffering and not be
able to help her. Throughout Chinese medical history, many
well-known practitioners started their medical career as a result
of their determination to cure their parents' illnesses. But this
was not true of me. I had never dreamed of being a doctor, for
the simple reason that I didn't like hospitals: the thought of
seeing people suffering every day put me off. During the
cultural revolution, even if I had wanted to be a doctor, it
would not have been possible, since we all had to go to the
countryside after graduation from high school, to be "re-educated" by peasants; we didn't have much choice for our future
careers.

I started to read herbal books when I was very young. Every
summer holiday, when I went to see my grandmother in the
countryside, I would sit in my grandfather's study for hours,
reading those old yellow coloured herbal books which had been
kept in my family for many years. The idea that those herbs
could cure almost everything, fascinated me. I tried to find out
which herbs could be used to treat a cold or a stomach ache, but
that was not my real interest; I read them because I hoped
that one day, when I went to the country to be "re-educated",
my knowledge of herbal medicine would be useful. It was
not until 1978, when the cultural revolution was over, that I
got the chance to go to university and choose my own future
career.

I actually wanted to be a writer, to write lovely stories, and
make people's lives better through the world of imagination. I
was a dreamer when I was a child, I liked to dream in the sleep-
less midsummer nights, looking into the dark blue sky with

thousands of twinkling stars, dreaming about the people who live on the moon, and concocting beautiful stories based on my dreams. But I was told that it was too dangerous to be a writer, because during the cultural revolution, nobody could write freely. Therefore most writers wrote rubbish, and were not respected. I was also told that I should not choose a career in politics, or a "cultural" career such as journalism or teaching. My parents persuaded me to choose herbal medicine as my career; to continue the "family business". During the cultural revolution, the red guards were encouraged to destroy almost anything that was old, belonging to the old culture. But luckily Chairman Mao was a great believer in traditional medicine, and said, "Traditional medicine is a great treasure trove; we must discover and develop it." The other reason I chose traditional medicine instead of modern (western) medicine was that herbal medicine is much safer to practise than modern medicine: herbal practitioners only feel the patient's pulse and prescribe herbal remedies. They don't have to "wield knives and guns", so do not see any bleeding and death, which is something that I hated even to think of before my medical career.

The first university I applied to was the Shanghai University of Traditional Chinese Medicine. Luckily, I passed the examination, left the countryside, and started the real "re-education" at the university many people would have loved to attend. Although I forced myself to study very hard, because I knew how lucky I was to have got a place there, I was only 17 years old, and had very little knowledge of traditional Chinese medicine. I soon realised that it was not as simple as I had imagined. The subjects which I was taught were so difficult to understand; for example, the Yin-Yang philosophy and the Five Elements theory. Whether or not we understood the ancient philosophy, we had to memorise it precisely, otherwise we would not pass our examinations. Worse than that was that we also had to study modern medicine at the same time! It made us extremely confused: we were told in the morning by a traditional doctor who taught us the basic theory of Traditional Chinese Medicine that the kidney takes charge of both the urinary and reproductive functions; it has its specific body opening in the ears; the condition of the kidney determines the condition of the bone; and it is the root of the life force, etc. But in the afternoon, we would have a lesson on human anatomy, and the western trained doctor would show us the real body and tell us where the kidneys are located, and how the urine or kidney stone would pass from the kidney through three narrow areas of ureter and pass out from the urethra. Not only could we not find any connection between the ears and the kidneys, but even the uterus which is located closest to the kidneys, does not share a single blood vessel with the kidneys! Which medicine is the better one? Which one actually cures illness?

One day I saw a short verse on a wall of a public lavatory in the university: "Studying traditional medicine in 1980s = analysing the antique in the atomic age!" Obviously there were many students like me, who felt frustrated and confused. Why should we still study these ancient remedies if we now have this wonderful modern medicine which explains everything so clearly, and scientifically?

Although this may have confused many others, it didn't bother me for long, coming as I do from a family which has a strong belief in traditional medicine. My uncle used to suffer from a chronic cough for years; he tried every cough medicine, antibiotics, but nothing worked, until one day he was recommended to see a famous TCM (Traditional Chinese Medicine) doctor. After a few days of taking the herbal tea which was prescribed by this doctor according to his TCM diagnosis, the cough stopped. My aunt used to practise herbal medicine and acupuncture to help the locals, when her university was moved to the countryside during the cultural revolution, and there was a lack of medical care. Through practising acupuncture and herbal medicine she saved many lives. Once she was called up in the middle of the night by a villager, to see a little boy with a severe nose bleed. With nothing but a few tiny needles she stopped the bleeding quickly. She gained a tremendous reputation in the area and was called "celestial being Xu".

My mother used to suffer from many chronic conditions such as palpitations, insomnia, headaches, asthma, enlarged liver, chronic nephritis, etc. Almost from top to toe no organs seemed to be healthy. Despite all the pills and tablets she took religiously every day, nothing really helped her. After her retirement, she had more time for herself and determined to sort out her own health problems. She realised that some of her symptoms were actually caused by the side effects of the drugs. Although she had taken herbal medicine from time to time, she had never been able to do it properly because she was too impatient to prepare the herbal medicine. Her general constitution had become very weak, and out of balance. So she started to take some herbal medicine prescribed by a TCM doctor in the winter to strengthen her lung *qi* (the immune system of the lungs), prevent the flu or common cold which often led to attacks of asthma and bronchitis. At the same time, she practised *Tai Chi* and *Qi Gong* (physical and meditative exercises) which also helped her to rebalance the disordered energy in her organs and enrich the vital *qi* (energy). A few years after her retirement, she gave up her "medicine bottle" completely, hardly had any cough in winter, and no more headaches or insomnia. TCM changed her life, so she not only strongly encouraged me to study TCM but also started her own research into *Qi Gong*. Eventually she set up a Qi Gong Institute in the town where she lives and travelled thousands of miles to visit many Qi Gong masters who live in other parts of China, including a few Taoists who live in the mountains far away from Shanghai. She has taught and helped lots of people, many of whom have now recovered from serious illnesses by practising *Qi Gong* like my mother herself did.

With great faith in Traditional Chinese Medicine, I studied very hard. Five years of study at the university soon passed; it was a bit like learning to drive. I had now passed the driving test; although I did not know how the car actually worked mechanically, I did know how to use it. Only after many years of practice, I am beginning to understand more and more of what I was taught at the university. I now feel like an experienced driver who has finally become a part of the car. In this book, I would like to share my knowledge and experience with anyone who is curious to know how Traditional Chinese Medicine works. I would also like to dedicate this book to all my patients. I sincerely hope this small book will give you the answers that I did not have enough time to give before.

Foreword

Atopic eczema is a major problem in northern Europe. Most people know someone who is affected, usually a child but also quite often an adult. The skin becomes inflamed and exceedingly itchy, as a result of which life can become a nightmare. Unfortunately, the treatments currently available from western medicine are of limited effectiveness; although most sufferers can be helped to a degree, the benefit often falls short of what is needed.

It was ten years ago that one of my eczematous patients first reported a near-miraculous response to herbal treatment prescribed by Dr Ding-Hui Luo, a Chinese doctor in London's Chinatown. I have been intrigued and impressed by Chinese herbal treatment ever since. I have been involved in research in collaboration with Dr Luo and, more recently, with Dr Xu, whose aim has been to demonstrate to me and to my colleagues in conventional medicine, using the scientific method, that Chinese herbal medicine can provide effective treatment for atopic eczema. Although we now know that this is certainly the case, we still do not understand how the herbs given to these sufferers so frequently provide such impressive benefits.

Of course, the herbs used by the Chinese contain pharmacological compounds which we would consider to be drugs, and many of these are already known to conventional medical science. Many of the herbs are identical or closely related to ones that were used by herbalists in Europe before the demise of herbal medicine here earlier this century. However, the many hundreds of herbs used by the Chinese are very likely to contain other compounds which are not yet known in the West and which may help patients with a wide variety of diseases.

While we in the West have tended to focus on treatments that consist of a single pharmacological compound, the norm in Traditional Chinese Medicine is to prescribe mixtures of several herbs each of which would not work as well on its own. Many of us in western medicine believe that it is time to re-explore this more complex approach, which may maximise the benefit of particular compounds while minimising side effects.

Increased awareness of the therapeutic potential of Chinese medicinal herbs is providing a new stimulus in western medicine, and a new perspective. I would like to see Chinese herbal medicine more readily available to patients in the West, and more readily available to researchers who wish to understand more clearly how it works. I believe that there will be mutual advantage in collaboration between the Chinese and western traditions.

I met Guang Xu several years ago, and was immediately impressed by her ability, her energy and her charm. She has a well-developed understanding of western medicine, which gives her unusual insight into the problems that underlie Traditional Chinese Medicine. She is therefore well equipped to provide readers with a "feel" for these principles, and I am delighted that she responded to my encouragement to write this book, despite the great linguistic difficulties involved.

Dr David Atherton FRCP,
Consultant in Paediatric Dermatology,
Great Ormond Street Hospital for Children,
London WC1N 3JH.

Introduction
– Medicine or miracle?

Mankind now has the ability to travel into space and land on the moon, yet we are still plagued with diseases that have afflicted the human race from time immemorial.

The Chinese have a saying: "The water can carry a boat, but can sink a boat too." In these modern times we suffer less from illness than our forefathers, but we suffer from many diseases that they had never even heard of.

Tuberculosis used to be one of the most fatal diseases ever to threaten man half a century ago, but now that it has been conquered, we still cannot relax: in its place we have HIV and AIDS. Eczema, one of the most common conditions in the world, still has no complete cure. Its incidence has increased by over 30% in the last 30 years. More than 10% of pupils in UK primary schools are asthmatic. It is said that this is a direct result of increasing pollution in our living environment.

Food is subject to the same concerns. To grow food faster, and keep it fresh for longer, most of our food is now full of chemicals. So more and more people are buying food which is labelled "organic". While we are already suffering from diseases caused by unhealthy food and a polluted environment, we do not want to take poisoning medicines that are supposed to cure us, do we?

People now want quality of life, not just for survival. Female patients would rather have their hormones rebalanced than have their wombs removed.

Although modern medicine has been successful in conquering many illnesses that humans have suffered for centuries, more and more people are turning to traditional cures ("alternative" or "complementary" medicine). Used together, these disciplines can offer even greater scope to conquer disease, improve the quality of our life and enable us to enjoy it more.

China's healing method is based on natural herbs, acupuncture, meditation, massage, food therapy, and a completely different perspective on treatment from that of the West. Collectively, it's called TCM, Traditional Chinese Medicine.

Traditional Chinese Medicine has, in fact, been practised outside China for many years, since the first groups of Chinese people emigrated. But most Chinese doctors practised in herbal shops located in various "Chinatowns"; in Chinese, these practitioners were called *zuo tang yi sheng* (the doctor who sits in a shop). Inevitably, their patients were almost all Chinese. There are now many practitioners in big cities in the USA, Far Eastern countries and almost any country that has a Chinatown.

Today more and more British people are seeking Chinese herbal treatments, especially for skin diseases such as eczema. Almost any family that has a member suffering from eczema now knows that Chinese herbs can help.

Traditional Chinese Medicine is not only an art of healing, but is also an art of being well. Yin-Yang philosophy is an ancient philosophy that applies not only to medicine, but also to the environment in which we are living. Although most people start to seek medication only when they are really sick, health is not just not taking any medication.

According to ancient Chinese philosophy, healthy and ill are two aspects of one thing: the balance of Yin and Yang. When the Yin and the Yang in our body or organs are balanced, we are healthy, but the Yin and Yang in our body are never stable, because we live in such a complicated world. The climate changes all the time, our moods change every day, we travel a lot, we eat different foods in different seasons. So the Yin and Yang aspects in our body change. How we can keep them balanced is the Chinese art of healing and being well.

Chinese herbal medicine has become more and more popular in Britain over the last few years, there are now schools that teach Traditional Chinese Medicine and books about Chinese herbal medicine, but they tend to be aimed at the practitioners rather than the people who are taking herbal medicine. There are very few books that answer their questions. This is what I am setting out to do.

Since I came to work in London in 1989, I have seen many patients with many different complaints. I am astonished at how enthusiastic my patients are about the traditional medicine from the Far East: many of them are curious about what I prescribe for them and want to know how it works and why.

To help my patients to understand the medicine that they are taking, and enable them to get the most benefit from it, in this small book I will explain as simply as possible the basic theory of TCM. Once they understand the ancient healing art, they will know how to maintain their health after the treatment.

During treatment, I often give my patients advice on their diet according to our tradition. In China, food and medicine are considered to "share the same source"; we regard most food as medicinal. Herbs form part of our daily food. So, while a patient is taking herbal medicine, his diet is very important. Even after the treatment, keeping to the right diet will also help to prevent the illness from recurring. For people who are healthy, but would like to be healthier, maintain well being and prevent illness, this knowledge will also be of use.

What is Traditional Chinese Medicine?

Most people who have heard of or experienced Traditional Chinese Medicine have found it a bit mysterious.

How can a tiny needle have such a magical effect, or a bunch of dry herbs cure a disease which people have suffered from for years? How can a practitioner make his diagnosis just by looking at the patient's tongue and feeling the pulse, without X-ray or blood test? It is not based on scientific evidence, but Yin and Yang philosophy. It is like a religion; we believe it, but there is no explanation for it.

Since traditional medicine is rooted in the culture of centuries, it cannot be easily explained or measured by modern scientific language and methods. Without a total understanding of its background and its history, it is very difficult to understand.

As a child living in China in a family with a long connection with traditional medicine, I heard lots of mysterious stories about it.

One story that fascinated me for a long time in my childhood was about pulse reading. A famous doctor was asked to go to the forbidden city to see one of the emperor's favourite concubines who was suffering from a life-threatening disease. It has always been said that a highly skilled doctor should be able to make a diagnosis "without any hint from the patient" (*Bing jia bu yong kai kou* – the patients do not need to open their mouths). Although he was asked to "see" the patient, the doctor was only allowed to "see" the patient with a traditional silk screen between them, so he could not see her at all. Pulse reading is regarded as one of the most important diagnostic methods in Chinese medicine. So, the only thing he was allowed to do was to take her pulse, but without touching her. But how could he do this? The clever doctor showed the emperor his magical skill by feeling the pulse through a silk thread, one end of which was held by the doctor's fingertips and the other end bound to the patient's wrist. A herbal medicine was soon prescribed by the doctor, and after a few days of treatment the concubine recovered from the illness. There are lots of stories like this that have been passed on from generation to generation.

In China traditional medical skill was based on experience. People would be expected just to copy this treatment without question. If one formula worked for one patient, when another patient had the same condition, exactly the same formula would be used. This could cause problems. For instance, someone might have got a prescription containing ingredients like "a pair of crickets", but "they must be the original pair, not re-paired ones", so divorce was not recognised even for crickets! Or: "This prescription must be cooked with the water of melted snow from New Year's Day." It was difficult to prove which cures were accidental and which were not in those days.

Not until I started to study at the Shanghai University of Traditional Chinese Medicine did I begin to understand it.

One day, I asked my teacher who taught us pulse reading whether he had ever heard the story about the doctor who took the patient's pulse via a silk thread. He laughed at first, then said that it was a true story, but in his opinion what the emperor's mistress was suffering from was a kind of acute communicable disease which many others were suffering at the time, so the doctor gathered the information from her family, found her symptoms were very similar to the others, and prescribed a formula according to his instinctive sense. It was pure guesswork! Otherwise he would have been executed .

I also remember that, when I first started to study TCM, a patient who suffered from a chronic infection after an operation for appendicitis was sent to one of the training hospitals of the university. Professor Xia, the consultant dermatologist of TCM at the hospital, examined him, and found that the wound caused by the operation about three years ago was still wide open with a lot of pus and dark blood. Since the chronic infection, a fistula had formed on his lower right abdominal wall. Despite treatment with the strongest antibiotics and several more operations to remove the fistula, it kept re-forming. Professor Xia treated his wound carefully with his bare hands using some unsterilised herbal powder from an unsterilised bowl. A few days later the wound started to heal. It got smaller and smaller each day, and the red inflamed skin surrounding the wound started to show some normal colour. After a few weeks the wound was completely healed! So, why did the patient who suffered from chronic infection not respond to antibiotics, but did respond to unsterilised herbal powder?

Professor Xia had a good explanation for it. He quoted from the first medical book of TCM (The Canon of Interior Medicine [Huang Di's *Nei Jing*]): "If the vital *qi* is strong enough inside [the body], no evil *qi* can disturb it [the body]; the place where the evil *qi* gathers is the area that lacks vital *qi*." According to his diagnosis, this particular patient's *qi* (vital energy or immune system) was not strong enough in the first place, probably before the illness, and the long period of suffering and different unsuccessful treatments had made it even worse. The evil *qi* (infection) lingers for a long time if the vital *qi* is weak. So, two different ranks of herbs were required in the prescription for this particular patient. Professor Xia stressed that tonic herbs were needed to build up the patient's resistance to fight the external pathological factors, and also herbs to dissipate heat and detoxify the body. He called this treatment "combating poison with poison". The poison was strong, but it was used externally, so would not harm the vital *qi* inside. The causes of the illness were not only the evil *qi* itself, but also the weak vital *qi*. This treatment is called *Fu Zheng Qu Xie* (reinforcing body resistance to eliminate pathogens). It was not Professor Xia's invention, but has been used for thousands of years!

TCM is obviously not based on science, for my Chinese forefathers lived several thousand of years ago without microscopes, X-ray machines, antibiotics or any of the paraphernalia of scientific medicine.

It is said that a microscope is the prolonged sight of a human being, and that science is the history of human beings trying to prolong their arms, legs and sight. We invented the telephone because we wanted to send our voices as far as possible. We invented the spaceship because we wanted to go as far as possible. But 5,000 years ago, when we didn't have any of these inventions the only thing that ancient Chinese people could do was use their five sense organs and brain to observe and analyse the causes of illness, to find some truth about how the body works, how herbs work, how diseases develop, and the relationship between them. After using ourselves as guinea pigs for generations, we developed our own special system of medical theory.

Our forefathers invented paper, gunpowder, the compass, mobile printing blocks, silk, etc. with no knowledge of how and why they worked from a scientific point of view. They invented these things using their rich imagination and instinctive practical experience. As long as it works, why question it?

In many cases modern science still cannot explain how and why traditional medicine works. Just like a child learning to speak, as long as their words can express their feelings or needs, we would not criticise their grammar. If we all have to study grammar before we speak our first word, human beings would have to suffer even more.

It is not always easy to prove a fact scientifically, yet sometimes we can tell a truth by intuition. To explain how Chinese doctors discover the right treatment and how to make the right diagnoses, the "black box theory" may help.

Suppose there is a black box containing some coloured powder in it, but we don't know what colour it is and we are not allowed to look inside. We want to find out what is in it, so what can we do? Well, firstly we could give it a signal, and see how it responds. For instance, we could put another different coloured powder into the box and see what happens. If say, we put blue into the box, and it comes out green, we would know that the other in the box is yellow. A few thousand years ago, the human body was like a "black box" for Chinese doctors. Dissection was considered immoral in China, so they were not able to study anatomy or analyse the structure of the human body. They had to use their brains to analyse diseases.

There is a story about Zhang Zhong Jing, the famous Chinese medical saint, which gives us some idea about how difficult it was. (His important contribution to TCM is described in Chapter 3.) He lived about 1,700 years ago, and when an acute communicable disease killed thousands of people in the town where he lived, lots of them were buried in the field. When some of the bodies were dug out by wild dogs or wolves, he got a chance to see real human organs. But even though he knew where the organs were located in the human body, without a microscope, he still could not find out about the structure and function of these organs. So most physicians simply used their own bodies as a "black box", treating themselves with herbal medicines. By trial and error and feedback from the human body, they found out the effects of herbs on the body.

Traditional Chinese Medicine has always been strongly   influenced by the ancient Yin-Yang philosophy and the theory of the Five Elements. Since the philosophy and the theory are so ancient and abstruse, many people find them rather mysterious and difficult to understand, but, in fact, they are very simple ideas which will be explained in more detail in Chapter 3.

TCM is a complete discipline that deals with human physiology, pathology, diagnosis, and prevention of diseases. It has built up a specific, integrated system of theory over the centuries, rich in clinical experience: an important constituent of the Chinese cultural treasure-trove, TCM has distilled the experiences of the Chinese people in their long struggle against disease, evolving into a particular system of medical theory through long-term clinical practice under the influence and direction of ancient insights and philosophies.

———————————— 2 ————————————

A brief 5,000-year history

Sheng Nong – the first person in Chinese history who tasted "poison plants"

It is said that traditional Chinese medicine has a history going back 5,000 years to the time of Sheng Nong, a divine husband-man (also said to be the first emperor). He was born around about 3500 B.C.

The unrecorded history of using plants to treat and prevent illness in China goes back much further than a few thousand years. Our ancestors must have used natural herbs as healing materials since the first group of the Han race lived by the Yellow River. Unfortunately, most of their practical experiences have been lost since we only have a few thousands of years of written records.

The earliest Chinese history book, *Shi Ji* (The Historical Records), written by Shi Ma Xian, first recorded the story of Sheng Nong. In his book he said, "Sheng Nong tasted various herbs and determined their medical property and value". Another historical writer, Liou Shu, wrote in his book *Tong Jan Wai Ji* (Historical Legends), "When ancient people suffered from diseases, no therapeutic medicine was known. Therefore the Emperor Yen (Sheng Nong) began to taste various herbs, and even encountered seventy species of poisonous ones in a day."

Sheng Nong identified the therapeutic value of herbs in a time prior to Chinese written history, so his achievements were handed down verbally to following generations. Although the stories about him might not be entirely accurate, certainly more than one person tasted these herbs – perhaps at the command of Sheng Nong!

Traditional Chinese medicine determines the effectiveness of a medicinal herb, firstly by taste, then its Yin and Yang nature (hot and cold property) and so on. Before giving herbal remedies to patients, our forefathers discovered the effectiveness of the herbs by tasting and testing them hundreds and thousands of times on themselves and certainly not on guinea pigs!

Huang Di (475 B.C.)

The history of human beings using medicinal herbs can be traced back to the Stone Age. We know that some animals instinctively pick certain leaves or herbs to eat when they are ill; just as some women would crave citrus fruit or other foods when they are pregnant!

In fact, our bodies give out signals all the time to inform us not only of what to take, but also when to take it. Our stomach rumbles when we are hungry; we yawn when we are tired. Most of us would only notice the most significant signals, but ignore or fail to notice many others.

Huang Di observed these signals very carefully to enable him to make accurate diagnoses for treatment with herbs. *Nei Jing* (Huang Di's Canon of Interior Medicine) is an excellent example of this wisdom. It incorporates the Yin-Yang philosophy, and a wealth of practical knowledge from his clinical observations.

Nei Jing is one of the oldest and certainly the most important existing Chinese medical textbook. It takes the form of the dialogue between the legendary Yellow Emperor and his minister Qi Bo on the topic of medicine. Even now, 2,500 years later, it is still regarded as one of the most important TCM textbooks to be used in medical school in China for the study of the fundamental theory of traditional Chinese medicine. It was said that "no one can be a good doctor without understanding *Nei Jing*".

Apart from the philosophical theory of Yin and Yang, and a description of the theory of the Five Elements, the contents of the book are unique. It includes physiology, pathology, therapeutics, classification of diseases and systems of meridians. Although, in the last two and half thousand years, many generations of physicians have enriched the theory of TCM with their clinical experiences, the principles and fundamental theory of TCM have not changed since *Nei Jing*. As one person commented: "All we have done after *Nei Jing* is try to explain the complicated clinical phenomena of illness and health of the human body, using the Yin-Yang philosophy and Five Elements theory from *Nei Jing*." This may not be a hundred per cent true, but the Yin-Yang philosophy and Five Elements theory have always been considered the most important essence of traditional Chinese medicine. They were first mentioned and used in *Nei Jing*.

The most important principles of Chinese medicine are still based on the theories which *Nei Jing* first described. The most significant are as follows:

The concept of holism

When *Nei Jing* was published, Huang Di knew that the human body was composed of a variety of tissues and organs, each performing a particular function, and each a component part of the activities of the whole body. The human body is an integral whole in that its constituent parts are inseparable in structure, connected with and conditioned by one another in physiology, and interacting with one another in pathology.

"The lungs connected with the skin and their condition reflected on vellus hairs; the nose is as the window of the lungs . . . ."

This may sound peculiar, but let's have a close look at some of the most common conditions. For example, eczema (here I refer to atopic dermatitis), asthma and hay fever (or allergic rhinitis) are some of the most common conditions in this country. Although these three conditions affect different parts of the body (the skin, the lungs, the nose), and have very different symptoms (itchy skin, wheeziness or shortage of breath, running or blocked nose), modern medicine has now proved that they have similar causes: they are all considered to be allergic conditions, and the allergy sources could be in the air (pollen breathed in through the nose), in food, or in the environment. Quite a number of people who suffer from eczema also suffer from hay fever or asthma, or both, since their causes are similar. In modern medicine, all these three conditions can be treated by the same drug. For instance, Becotide, a kind of steroid originally used to treat asthma, coincidentally made some patients' eczema better, and is now also used to treat eczema. Although the form of the drug can be different (oral tablet, inhaler, or ointment) the similarity in treatment was only discovered recently.

According to TCM theory, if we can improve the condition of the lungs, the skin condition will also improve, and vice versa.

So it is not surprising that the treatment of skin conditions with TCM involves some of the herbs normally used to "clear the heat from the lungs"!

"The universe and the human being form one holism." Man's close connection with nature is manifested by the fact that nature provides conditions indispensable to man's survival and whose changes may influence the human body directly or indirectly, thereby causing its corresponding responses. For example, taking the pulse is a very important way of making a diagnosis. This is determined not only by the individual person (their body size, their sex, their age), but also by the time of day and season of the year. For instance, during the day, your pulse could be relatively stronger and faster than at night; and pulses are more slippery and superficial in the spring and summer, and deeper in the winter.

Yin-Yang philosophy

In ancient Chinese philosophy, Yin and Yang are two opposite categories. At first, their connotations were quite simple, meaning turning away from and facing the sunlight respectively. The character of Yin has a symbol of the moon on the right side, which means overcast, or no sunshine, and the character of Yang has a symbol of the sun, which means bright, or the sun. But Yin and Yang have gradually been extended to describe any two opposite forces in nature. For example, hot or cold, down or up, right or left, internal or external, moving or static, and so on. Because they are opposites, the balance between them is vital. Yin and Yang can be used to express the basic aspects of anything. In *Nei Jing*, Huang Di used Yin and Yang to explain medical phenomena.

For instance, in the physiology section of *Nei Jing*, the surface of the human body is described as Yang, and the internal organs as Yin. Likewise, the back of the body is Yang and front of the body is Yin. There are eleven main organs in the body: five Zang organs (liver, kidney, spleen, lungs and heart), representing the characteristics of Yin; and six Fu organs (stomach, gallbladder, urinary bladder, large intestine, small intestine, and Sanjiao triple burner) which have Yang characteristics. The Sanjiao describes the three body cavities. The upper cavity is the area around the heart and lungs; the middle cavity is the area around the spleen and stomach; and the lower cavity is the area around the kidneys, liver, intestines and bladder. For making diagnoses, *Nei Jing* says: "If the person is a good doctor, he must be able to distinguish the signs of Yin and Yang first, by observing the complexion and taking the pulse." For treatment, *Nei Jing* recommends: "to treat a cold condition, a medicine with a warm nature should be used; to treat a hot condition, a medicine with a cold nature must be used." These ancient principles still form the basis of TCM, after 2,500 years!

But Yin and Yang theory alone cannot explain everything in medicine, since the relationships between man and nature, diseases and organs are very complicated. The Five Elements theory also plays an important role.

Five Elements theory

The Five Elements (Earth, Fire, Water, Metal and Wood) are regarded as aspects of character. Each element rules different internal organs, parts of the body, emotional expressions, colours, taste and energies, so before making a diagnosis and formulating a prescription, the herbalist needs to know which element most closely represents the patient's character. For example, each types are prone to water retention, indigestion and muscular tenderness.

Meridians

The doctrine of meridian, or the theory of channels and collateral, deals with the physiological functions and pathological changes in the circulatory system and the channels' relationship with the Zang Fu organs. It is an important component of the theoretical system of TCM. Twelve meridians were described in *Nei Jing*, and each meridian is named after one of the body's organs.

The idea of the prevention of disease

Modern medicine now seeks to prevent disease rather than just to cure it. This philosophical imperative had already been expounded in *Nei Jing*: Huang Di wrote: "The superior doctor is one who can successfully check diseases before they have developed." "If healthy energy (the resistance of the human body to diseases) is there (inside the human body), evil (evil factors affecting health) cannot harm it (the human body)." This theory became one of the essential principles of traditional Chinese medicine. Medical students are still told to strengthen the body's vital energy during and after treatment. For example, to treat cancer, patients are quite often given tonic herbs as well as herbs to combat the poisons (the cancer itself). In winter, everything in nature is in a restoration phase, so winter is the time to take tonic herbs, in order to rebalance vital energy and prevent illness in the spring.

Hua Tuo

Hua Tuo (born around 1,700 years ago) was a famous doctor in the East Han dynasty. He specialised in surgical diseases and created a famous herbal formula – *Ma Fei San* – which he used for general anaesthesia during operations to remove matter from the abdominal cavity. Sadly, the formula of Ma Fei San has been lost. But, what has come down from him is the origin of the important relationship between exercise and good health.

Hua Tuo believed that "running water would never be rotten, nor would the pivot of a door ever be moth-eaten". The same is true of the human body: regular exercise keeps us healthy. He invented the five styles of Chinese boxing. These started as exercises imitating the movements of five different animals: the tiger, deer, bear, monkey and bird, and have evolved into Tai Chi.

Zhang Zhong Jing

Regarded as the saint of Chinese herbal medicine, Zhang Zhong Jing was born in the Latter Han Dynasty (A.D. 142–220). He established the Chinese formula therapy (the principles or rules of forming a prescription) and invented therapeutic rules: *Bian Zheng Lueng Zhi* – diagnosis and treatment based on an overall analysis of symptoms and signs and the patient's physical condition. His therapy was to divide all signs and symptoms into six stages (three Yin and three Yang). He used *Si Zheng*, the "four diagnoses" method, based on observation, auscultation, olfaction, pulse taking and palpation to examine the existing systems.

Born in He Nan province, he was a very talented and hardworking man of precise judgement. Even as a youth, it was said that "he was very meditative and humble, and intended to become a famous medical practitioner".

A plague was raging when he was in Chin-Chou (a city in He Nan): having witnessed the death of about two-thirds of his 200-odd relatives, he became determined to study medicine. Having done so, he completed the immortal 16 volumes of *Shang Han Za Bing Luen* (Treatise on Fevers and Miscellaneous Diseases).

Shang Han Za Bing Luen was later edited by Dr Wang Su-He into two volumes: *Shang Han Luen* and *Jig Gui Yao Lu*. *Shang Han Luen* deals with infections, contagious and epidemic fevers, while *Jig Gui Yao Lu* deals with other diseases of the digestive, respiratory, urological and nervous systems; metabolism, gynaecology, etc.

Li Shi Zheng

Li Shi Zheng (1518–1593), the greatest naturalist in Chinese history, was kind, willing to help all, and did not collect fees for his treatment. His medical ability was soon widely recognised. Later, he assumed the position of chief court physician on the recommendation of the mother of the oldest son of a prince whom he had cured from spontaneous coma of undetermined origin. Li subsequently served in the Imperial Academy of Medicine in the capital. Ill health prompted him to retire from these pressures and responsibilities and he thereafter returned home to study and write.

Li's fame is due to a work that took him 40 years to complete. Li Shi Zheng's "General Catalogue of Herbs" (*Beng Cao Gang Mu*) was one of the most outstanding books of its time and remains an important reference for all those interested in Chinese medicine. Beginning at the age of 30, his treatise went through three revisions before its final conclusion in 1578 in his seventieth year. Unfortunately, Li never lived to see his monumental efforts published due to difficulties in printing arrangements. When it finally appeared in 1596 through the press of Qian Long in Nanking, it became an instant success. This monumental publication consisted of 52 volumes with 1,160 illustrations.

The early influence of western medicine and the setting up of a medical school

During Li's time, the Ming Dynasty (1368–1644), the Roman Catholic Church initiated missionary activity in China. Matteo Ricci was one of the first to arrive in 1580 followed by Nicholas Longobardi, Alphonso Vagnoni, and Francisco Sambiaso. They introduced European scientific knowledge to China and translated many books on science and medicine into Chinese.

The Protestant Church did not send its emissaries to China until the Ching Dynasty (1644–1911). These included men with medical training, such as a British doctor called Colledge and an American doctor, Lockhart, who did much to implant western medicine into China in the nineteenth century. Their activities usually began in Hong Kong, Macao and Canton, gradually extending to the interior.

For thousands of years, Chinese doctors passed their medical knowledge on privately, through family members. Because of the numerous civil wars, the government wasn't able to set up a national medical school until about 1,000 years ago, in the Song Dynasty (960–1368). According to historical records, the school had nine different departments, including: the department of internal medicine (*Da Fang Mai*), the department of infectious diseases (*Feng Ke*), the department of paediatrics (*Xiao Fang Mai*), the department of surgery and dermatology (*Chang Zhong Zhe Sang*), the department of ophthalmology (*Yan Ke*), the department of obstetrics (*Chan Ke*) and the department of acupuncture. After examinations in local towns 300 students attended the school. After studying many classic medical books, they had to treat the soldiers in the army, and write case histories, as part of their training. In about 1076, Dr Wang Wei Yi, a medical expert and a court physician of the northern Song Dynasty, created two bronze models of men marked with the 12 meridians and 354 acupuncture points. They were used as teaching aids at the school. All the acupuncture points were filled with water and then covered with wax; when the students punctured the right points, water would come out through the wax. One was lost in Shan-yan in the southern Song Dynasty; the other is now displayed in the National Tokyo Museum, Japan.

In 1919 the first modern Chinese medical college (now the Shanghai University of Traditional Chinese Medicine) was set up in Shanghai.

In 1929, doctors returning from Japan, where they had received their medical degrees, recommended the abolition of Traditional Chinese Medicine. Fortunately for the practitioners of TCM (and the University) the proposal was rejected at a national medical assembly held in Shanghai on 17 March, 1929.

Traditional Chinese Medicine in modern China

In China we talk about "Chinese medicine" and "western medicine". Almost all modern medical hospitals have a TCM department and, conversely, TCM hospitals have modern medical departments. The patients may choose.

At TCM medical schools, apart from studying ancient Chinese, students also have to study some modern medicine such as physiology, pathology, biochemistry, human anatomy, pharmacology, etc. Quite a lot of doctors who have had modern medical training decide after several years of practice to study traditional medicine. Then they might practise both disciplines to get optimum results.

Both types of medicine have their advantages and disadvantages. For instance, in the treatment of cancer, although many types of cancer can be cured by means of operations, radiotherapy or chemotherapy, because the treatment is so harsh, if the patient's general constitution is weak, he will not be able to tolerate the treatment. With herbal medicine, we can not only increase the effectiveness of the treatment, but also build up the immune system, and reduce the side effects from the drugs or the therapy. Even in terminal cases, patients can live much longer and the quality of their remaining life be improved.

3

The philosophy and theory of Yin-Yang and the Five Elements

The various branches of TCM, such as herbal medicine, acupuncture, Qi Gong, massage (Chinese Osteopathy) and food therapy all share the same philosophy and theory: Yin-Yang and the Five Elements.

Yin-Yang

Yin means "the moon" or "overcast"; the Chinese character of Yin contains a symbol of the moon. Yang means "the sun", or "sunshine", so the Chinese character of Yang has a symbol of the sun. Yin represents the dark and cold nature of any object, while Yang symbolises the bright and warm nature. Since a place which faces the sun is always on the south side of a mountain, and a place backing the sun is always on the north side, so Yin and Yang can also be interpreted as north and south. Many places in China are named after Yin and Yang. For example, "Shan Yin", "Huai Yin", and "Xiang Yang", "Luo Yang", etc. They mean: north side of the mountain, north side of the river Huai; and the south side of the mountain, south side of the river Huai. Yin also means negative, while Yang means positive. For example, a positive ion, is called "Yang ion", and a negative ion is called "Yin ion".

Weather forecasting

Originally, the people who believed in the Yin-Yang theory were called *Yin-Yang Jia* (Yin-Yangists). In *Han Shu, Yi Wen Zhi* (the

Book of Han – History of Art and Culture), it says that the Yin-Yang theory was initiated by Qi He. Qi He was known in Yao time (3000 B.C?) as an astrologer and a weatherman. Another book *Shang Shu, Yao Dian* (Shang Book, the History of Yao) said that Emperor Yao ordered Qi to observe the sky, the sun, the moon, and the stars, in order to tell people the time.

So the words Yin-Yang were probably first used in connection with weather forecasting and the relationship between day and night, warm and cold, sunny and cloudy, etc. Since the weather played a vital role in agriculture, observing the sky was a very important job.

The Yin-Yangists not only observed the weather patterns and the changing of seasons in order to apply some logic to them, but also nature as a whole. They then applied the logic they had discovered in nature to human beings and to the relationship between nature and human beings. For instance, they might have used it to predict a change of dynasty. So, the influence of Yin-Yang can be seen in other cultures as well as that of medicine.

Some Chinese people still believe not only that human actions have a huge impact on nature, but that changes in nature can also influence human actions, such as in the sphere of politics.

Take the momentous events of 1975–76. In August 1975, in the Tang-Shan area, less than 100 miles from Peking, there was a severe earthquake, which killed more than half of the citizens of the city of Tang-Shan. It was one of the most severe earthquakes in China's entire history. Some Chinese astrologists believed it to be the sign of a changing dynasty, and predicted Chairman Mao's fall. Sure enough, in December 1975, Zhu De died; then in January 1976 Zhou En-Lai died of cancer; and on 9 September 1976, Chairman Mao also died. Was this just coincidence?

The Yin-Yangists eventually applied their logic to Chinese medicine, to explain human physiology, pathology and the nature of herbs, etc. For instance, in *Nei Jing*, the earliest Chinese medical textbook, this logic was used to explain human physiology: "The sky is light and bright, the earth is dark and heavy; invisible matter rising from the earth forms the clouds; invisible matter going down from the sky becomes the rain. Therefore, the rain is from the earth, and the clouds are from the sky." The same logic was applied to the human body: "The air is light, therefore it goes out from the holes on the top; the water is heavy, therefore it goes out from the holes at the bottom." "The sky is round, and the earth is square; in the human body, the head is round and the feet are square." "There are both sun and moon in the sky; therefore we have two eyes; . . . there is wind and rain in the sky; we have happy and sad moods; the sky has thunder; we have a voice; . . . nature has summer and winter; we have fever and colds . . . . "

Philosophy

Yin and Yang are the two fundamental principles or forces in the universe, ever opposing and supplementing each other. Basically, Yang symbolises the more immaterial, bright, upward, positive states of matter, whereas Yin symbolises the more material, dark, downward, negative states of matter. The Yin and the Yang are the two stages of transformation.

The ancient Chinese considered almost everything in the universe to consist of opposites. For instance, up and down, left and right, hot and cold, sunny and cloudy, etc. Although opposites, they are very closely related to each other. Without Yang, Yin would have nothing to compare itself with, so would lose its meaning. Dark only has meaning when compared with light. The relationship between the front and the back is another good example. A book has a front cover and a back cover but, if the book only had one page, there would be no division between them; the front and the back would form one page. Therefore, the front and the back are the two stages of transformation; the front has to be compared with the one behind; if there was nothing behind, it would not be the front.

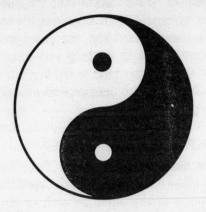

The Yin-Yang symbol

The Yin-Yang symbol is a good example of this concept. When you first look at it, you may have the impression that it is formed by two half "moons"; one black, and the other white. But the two "moons" seem to be moving; one is biting the other one's tail! They form a harmonious circle, like the symbol of a full moon. Although the two "moons" are completely different colours there is a white dot in the middle of the black "moon", and vice versa. Although the Yin-Yang symbol looks very simple and obvious, its meaning is very subtle. It displays the four aspects of the Yin-Yang relationship.

The opposition of Yin and Yang

Every phenomenon in nature has two opposite aspects or forces – Yin and Yang. These two opposite forces suppress each other to keep the opposite force under control. For instance, the summer and the winter are two opposite seasons, summer symbolises hot weather and winter symbolises cold weather; after the longest summer day, the winter season approaches slowly to suppress the hot weather, the days become shorter, and the nights become longer. The winter finally arrives with cold snow instead of fresh summer rain. Then, after the first thunder in spring, the warm weather slowly returns, suppressing the cold weather. We all know that the colour grey is the result of mixing white and black. Changing the balance of white or black can, however, affect the result: too much white will suppress the black and make the grey very light, and too much black will make the grey too dark, so although these two colours are opposites, they are also interdependent: both are equally necessary to form the grey colour.

The interdependence of Yin and Yang

So, although on the one hand Yin and Yang are two opposite aspects, on the other hand they are interdependent. Neither can exist independently of the other, so each of the two opposite aspects is the condition for the other's existence. Take day and night: the day is Yang and the night is Yin. If we were living in the dark all the time, we would not have any idea of the day, and without the day, the word night has no meaning. Just like up and down; if you compare the ground floor with the first floor, the first floor is up and the ground floor is down, but if the house only has one floor, although this is the ground floor, there is no reason to call it downstairs, since there is no upstairs. This relationship between Yin and Yang was described thus in *Nei Jing*: "Yin is inside, since the Yang is playing the role of the protector outside; the reason that Yang is outside, is because the Yin (that is inside) made it."

Mutual consumption of Yin and Yang

Although the Yin and Yang are two opposite forces always opposed to each other, the relationship between them is not static. In fact, the Yin and Yang are in a constant state of dynamic balance, which involves imbalance and rebalance. The imbalance of Yin and Yang can be seen in four different situations:

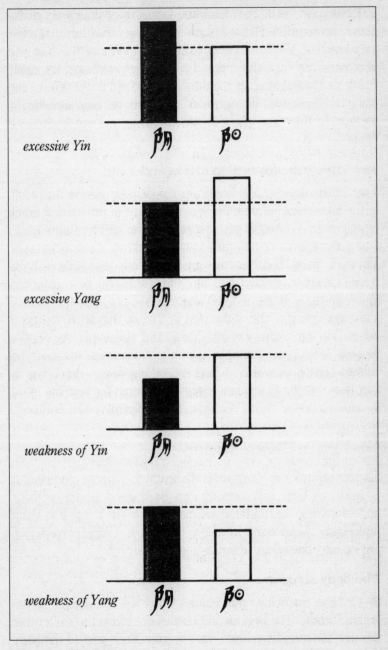

The imbalance of Yin and Yang

Either Yin is in the dominant position or Yang is in the dominant position. But there are two causes that can make the imbalance of Yin and Yang: if either the Yin or the Yang is weakened, its opposite side will be correspondingly stronger, breaking the balance; on the other hand, if either the Yin or the Yang is excessive, its opposite side will be correspondingly weaker. In this case, the Yin and the Yang are out of balance again.

The inter-transformation of Yin and Yang

The "imbalances" of Yin and Yang can also be seen as the result of the inter-transformation of Yin and Yang in different degrees or stages. In *Nei Jing*, it says: "excessive Yin will turn into Yang; and excessive Yang will turn into Yin." When the unbalance of Yin and Yang becomes too great, the opposite side will be forced to grow, so that the Yin and Yang will be rebalanced again. In the symbol of Yin-Yang, the Yin contains the seed of Yang and Yang contains the seed of Yin, so that when the need arises, Yin can transform into Yang, and vice versa. Again, the seasons are a good example: the hottest season is summer; the coldest season is winter, when everything seems dead, but in fact winter is the time when energy is restored for new life. As it is said in a poem: "With Winter here, can Spring be far behind?"

Yin-Yang in Chinese Medicine

The concept of Yin-Yang is fundamental to Chinese medicine. It is said in China that nobody can be a good doctor without understanding the fundamental meaning of Yin-Yang. Yin-Yang philosophy is evident in every aspect of Chinese medicine: physiology, pathology, diagnosis and treatment.

The body structure

In Chinese medicine, the human body is considered as an organic whole. The organs and tissues are related to each other through the meridians and vital energies. Each part of the body is also classified as Yin or Yang. For instance, the upper part of the body is Yang and the lower part is Yin; the surface of the body is Yang and inside the body is Yin; the front of the body is Yin and the back of the body is Yang. The Zang organs (lungs, kidneys, spleen, heart, liver) are Yin and the Fu organs (large intestine, small intestine, gallbladder, urinary bladder, stomach and triple burner [Sanjiao]) are Yang. However, these organs can be subdivided into Yin and Yang so that the heart and the lungs are Yang, and the kidneys, liver and spleen are Yin. A further subdivision means that the heart has the heart-Yin and heart-Yang, the lungs have the lung-Yin and the lung-Yang, etc.

In physiology

When the two Yin-Yang forces are in harmony, the person is healthy. The physiological function of the body Yang relies on the material basis of Yin, and Yang enriches Yin. If Yin and Yang are separated, the body dies. As it says in *Nei Jing*: "if the Yin is calm, and Yang is restored, the life activity will be in harmony; if the Yin and Yang are separated, the life activity stops."

In illness

In Chinese medicine illness is the result of a Yin-Yang imbalance. The immune system (*Zheng Qi* – where *Qi* is positive energy) has the Yin and the Yang two sides, as well as the exterior pathogenic factors, called the Yin-Evil and the Yang-Evil; if Yang-Evil invades the body it can cause excessive Yang and harm the Yin essence; symptoms of excessive heat will be seen. If the cause is Yin-Evil the cold symptoms will appear.

Diagnoses

In *Nei Jing*, it says that "the one who is good at making diagnoses would determine the character of Yin and Yang by taking the pulse and observing the complexion." Diagnosis is also made by analysis of differentiating pathological conditions in accordance with the *Ba Gang Bian Zheng* (eight principal syndromes). These eight syndromes are: external and internal; hot and cold; insufficiency and excessiveness; Yin and Yang.

Treatment

Since the cause of illness is Yin-Yang imbalance, the treatment is to balance the Yin-Yang with herbs, acupuncture, food, etc. "Hot" conditions should be treated with "cold" medicines while "cold" conditions should be treated with "hot" medicines. For excessive Yang, treat with Yin, for excessive Yin, treat with Yang. For Yang-deficient conditions, treat with Yang, for Yin-deficient conditions, treat with Ying, etc.

Five Elements (Wu Xing)

The original meaning of *Wu Xing* in Chinese is "five movements". The "five" refers to wood, fire, earth, metal and water. The "movement" describes the character of the five elements: how they move and change. For instance, a small seed in the soil (the earth) can become a big tree (wood); a fire can turn a wood to ash and form part of the earth. Even metal is not an isolated, or unchangeable object. For instance, iron can become rusty, and the rust will eventually also form part of the earth. When iron is heated to a certain temperature, it can also become fire, or even run like water. So, "movement" refers to the law of movement, or the law of changing within the five elements.

The Five Elements were first used in astrology. For instance, why was the Yellow Emperor (believed to be one of the earliest emperors in China's history) so called? Why wasn't he red or black? It is thought that the Han race developed on the bank of the Yellow River, and the reason that the river is yellow is because it runs through the famous "yellow-mud plateau", which makes the water yellow. The first year that the Yellow Emperor came to power, the astrologer predicted that the energy of the earth would be strong that year.

The Five Elements doctrine was used as a theoretical tool by ancient scholars to categorise everything in the universe. It is used in Traditional Chinese Medicine to explain the physiological and pathological relationship between the internal organs, and their relationship with the environment, the treatment and the property and the taste of the herbs.

To understand the Five Elements doctrine, one should also realise that the Five Elements doctrine and the Yin-Yang theory share the same logic. Like the Yin-Yang theory that divides everything in the world into Yin and Yang, the Five Elements doctrine divides all things into five different elements according to their different characteristics. Things in the same group can also supplement each other, like the theory of Yin-Yang. For instance, herbs that have a Yin nature can be used to treat a condition that is caused by Yin deficiency. For example, according to the Five Elements doctrine, taste can be classified as sweet, salty, sour, bitter and pungent. Each taste is assigned to an element. Equally, each of the Yin organs is assigned to an element. So, since both liver and the sour taste are in the wood category, sour-tasting herbs are considered good for the liver.

The properties of the Five Elements

The properties of the Five Elements are as follows:

1) Wood has the property of growing freely and unfolding
2) Fire has the property of warming and flaring up
3) Earth has the property of generating, transforming and receiving
4) Metal has the property of purifying and descending
5) Water has the property of nourishing and flowing downwards.

The interrelationships of the Five Elements

Interpromotion

Ancient Chinese scholars discovered a common phenomenon in the universe: that the relationship between one thing closely followed by another, or one thing positively influenced by another, is called a "mother and son" relationship, or "generation in five elements".

The order of generation of the Five Elements is: wood generates fire, fire generates earth, earth generates metal, metal generates water, and water, in turn, generates wood.

Restriction

In addition to the phenomenon of generation in nature, ancient Chinese scholars also realised that an opposite universal phenomenon exists in nature: one thing is often inhibited or restricted by another. This relationship can be called "restriction in five elements".

The order of restriction of the Five Elements is: wood restricts earth, earth restricts water, water restricts fire, fire restricts metal, and metal, in turn, restricts wood.

The generation and restriction of the Five Elements are equally important in any relationship. If there were no restriction, the growth would have no control, and the normal balanced harmony would be upset. Therefore the two movements, generation and restriction, are very important to ensure a normal relationship between things.

Xiang Cheng (encroachment) and Xiang Wu (violation)

Encroachment occurs when one element over-restricts another. For instance, if the *qi* (energy) of wood is too strong, and the energy of metal cannot restrict or interact with it, then the wood will overwhelm the earth. In Chinese medicine, this is seen as "liver-*qi* invading the spleen".

Violation occurs when one element restricts another which it should actually be restricted by. This is also called "reverse restriction". For instance, water should be restricted by earth; however, if the wood is excessively strong, instead of being restricted by metal, it "invades" the metal. In Chinese medicine the interpretation is that the liver-fire is invading the lungs and causing a dry cough with chest pains.

The Five Elements in Chinese Medicine

The Five Elements theory can be used to describe the function and the character of the organs. For instance, the liver has the characteristics of wood, with a tendency to grow and expand;

the heart has the characteristics of fire, by circulating the blood; the spleen has the characteristics of the earth, being a source of nurture, like the earth is for plants. The lungs have characteristics of metal, with a tendency to descend, the kidneys have the characteristics of water, descending and nourishing.

The Five Elements doctrine is also used in diagnoses and treatment.

4

The invisible scenery –
the organs, the vital
substances and the
meridians

The internal organs

The original meaning of *Zang* is "hide" or "store", since the
organs are "hiding" inside the body and cannot be seen. But
since the Chinese characters were simplified, *Zang* has come to
mean only "organ"; there is no sense of hiding any more. *Xiang*
means "manifestation", or "expression", and here refers mainly
to the outward physiological and pathological manifestations of
the human body. So, in Chinese medicine, *Zang Xiang* refers to
the theory that by observing the physiological and pathological
manifestations of the human body (both internal and external),
the interactions of its various viscera with the structures of the
body and the external environment, a diagnosis can be made.

Chinese medicine is rather like traditional Chinese art,
emphasising the spirit or the feeling rather than the physical
detail. Similarly, western medicine mirrors western art, emphasising the reality of the object; the light, the colour, the texture
of the clothing, etc.

The internal organs of Chinese medicine are not to be
confused with western medicine's similar-sounding organs.
Some of the organs described in western medicine do not even
exist in Chinese medicine and vice versa. For example, Sanjiao
(or triple burners, upper, middle and lower) are portions of the
body cavity.

About a century ago, when western medicine was first
introduced to China, many Chinese doctors were amazed at the

western picture of human anatomy. Compared with the rather vague description in *Nei Jing* of the location of human organs, the meridians and their functions, the western picture was much more accurate.

Respect for one's elders is one of the most important of Chinese ethics. This respect extends to the dead. To harm a dead body is considered extremely disrespectful. Therefore, it is and always has been very difficult to find a body to be dissected for medical purposes. So it was not possible to prove whether the description of the human organs in *Nei Jing* was correct. In any case, since Chinese doctors did not normally perform operations on patients (apart from minor operations for skin abscesses), there was no need for them to know exactly where the organs lay.

Zhang Jing-Yue, a well-known physician in the Ming Dynasty, said in his "Systematic Compilation of the Internal Medicine" (*Lei Jing*): "*Zang* implies storage . . . while *Xiang* suggests figure and appearance. Since organs are located within the body and their phase is observed from outside the body, these two characters *Zang* and *Xiang* put together, denote phase of viscera."

The western concept of internal organs is to see each organ only in its isolated material-anatomical aspect, whereas Chinese medicine sees each organ as a complex system encompassing not only its anatomical entity but also its corresponding emotion, tissue, sense organ, mental faculty, and so on. In Chinese medicine, one organ's function may affect another organ's function, which can seem very confusing from the western medicine point of view. For instance, the "transformation and transportation" of the spleen in Chinese medicine, is a bit like the function of the small intestine in western medicine, which not only absorbs the nutrients from the food, but also transports the waste to the large intestine to form the stool. Another example is the symptoms of "Liver-*qi* stagnation": pain in the upper-right abdomen, which may have nothing to do with the "western" liver, and everything to do with the "western" gallbladder.

Dr Zhu Pei Weng, from Canton, lived during the Qing Dynasty, and came from a medical family – his father and brother were both well-known TCM doctors. A student of both western medicine and Chinese medicine, he wrote: "I started studying medicine as a teenager, and I have been practising it for over 20 years now. I used to study western medicine too, and having the chance to see real organs in a western medical hospital, I found that the description of the organs and their function is different from that of Chinese medicine . . . both medicines have their rights and wrongs . . . basically, Chinese medicine is good at explaining the logic, while western medicine is adept in analysing the details . . . ."

In *Nei Jing* the major internal organs are divided into two groups, the Yin organs and the Yang organs. The five Yin organs (heart, liver, spleen, lungs, and kidneys) "restore the vital

A picture of organs in human body from Nei Jing.

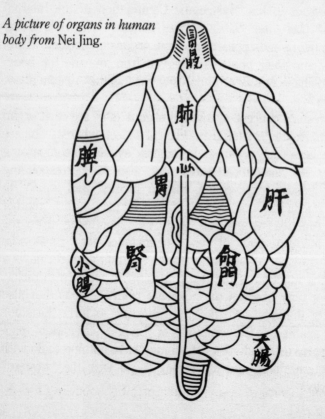

essence but do not pour it out; so it should be solid but not full";
the function of the six Fu organs (large intestine, small intestine,
gallbladder, urinary bladder, stomach and Sanjiao) is to "pass
the waste material but not restore it, so it should be full but not
solid." Compared with the five Yin (Zang) organs, the six Yang
(Fu) organs deal only with the "waste passages", therefore they
are only briefly described in Chinese medicine. Many of the
functions attributed to the six Yang (Fu) organs in western
medicine are attributed to the Yin (Zang) organs (lungs, kidneys,
spleen, heart, liver) in Chinese medicine. But this does not
mean that the six Yang (Fu) organs are not important; since
each organ's disorder will affect the others, particularly its
interrelated organ. To understand how this can happen is very
important for the purposes of clinical diagnosis and treatment.
Five of the Yang organs are introduced here, after their related
Yin organs.

The functions of the heart and the small intestine

In Chinese medicine, the heart is regarded as the most important
internal organ; it is called *Juen Zhu Zhi Guang* ("the master" or
the "emperor"). Its main functions are to govern blood and the
blood vessels, and to house the mind.

Governing blood

This refers to the fact that the heart has the function of "push-
ing" the blood along the blood vessels and is responsible for the
circulation of the blood, just as in western medicine. If the heart-
qi is profound, blood circulates freely in the blood vessels. The
condition of the heart can be found by taking the pulse and
observing the complexion: a red complexion mirrors the colour
of the heart and indicates that the heart-*qi* is profound; a pale
complexion indicates a deficiency of the heart-*qi* and blood. A
purple complexion indicates a stagnation of the blood.

Housing the mind

Chinese medicine holds that the heart is the residence of the
mind (*sheng*). *Sheng* has several interpretations, but in Chinese

medicine, it has just two meanings. In its narrow sense, *sheng* refers to the mind, the mental faculties. In its wider sense, *sheng* is used to indicate the general constitutional state of the mind, body and spirit. For example, when a patient's general constitution is poor, in the case of severe illness, for instance, his eyes can look dull. This is called "having no *sheng*". And if someone is sound in mind and body, it is called "having *sheng*".

Opening into the tongue

According to the theory of Traditional Chinese Medicine, each internal organ has a bond relationship with an external organ. "The heart opens into the tongue" means that the colour and the elasticity of the tongue indicate the state of the heart, so it is also said that the tongue is an "offshoot" of the heart.

So, if the heart houses the mind, the tongue should also be the "offshoot" of the mind. Our state of mind affects our speech, and we use our tongues to speak with, so tongues are linked in this way with speech. If the mind is clear, the speech will be clear. Take a look at a drunkard: his mind is muddled, and his tongue is slack. Therefore, stuttering and aphasia can indicate an abnormality in the state of the heart in Chinese medicine.

In the Five Elements theory, each organ is linked with a colour. Since the heart is a fire organ, its colour is red. If the heart has heat, the tip of the tongue turns redder, instead of its normal pink colour.

The small intestine and the heart are said to be interior-exterior related, since their channels are interrelated. The main function of the small intestine is that of receiving and transforming food; separating the useful substances from the waste (or the "clear" ones – the urine and the refined nutritious substances – from the "turbid" ones – the stool). Pathologically, this interrelationship between the small intestine and the heart can be seen when high blood pressure, caused by excessive fire in the heart, is transferred to the small intestine, causing a burning sensation during urination, and a red tongue tip, etc.

The functions of the liver and the gallbladder

In Chinese medicine the liver's functions differ from the liver's functions of western medicine. The most obvious difference is that in Chinese medicine, the liver's condition not only affects the digestive system, but also the emotions and the reproductive system. Therefore, many gynaecological disorders can be treated by restoring liver-*qi*.

The characteristics of the liver are also quite different even from the other four Yin organs in Chinese medicine. The liver is said to be an "army general", since its functions and disorder patterns reflect the characteristics of an army general. Chinese army generals are moody and can "catch fire" easily. The Chinese phrase "liver fire rising" means losing your temper. Although the liver is a Yin organ, it has lots of Yang or "male" characteristics. Even when its disorder pattern is caused by deficiency, it still often shows the signs of hyper-activity (hyper-activity of Yang caused by deficiency of Yin). It is said that "the liver Yin and blood are often deficient, while the liver Yang and liver-*qi* are always over-active." It is true that there are no patterns in Chinese medicine named as "liver Yang deficiency, or liver-*qi* deficiency"; since the liver Yang or liver-*qi* are never deficient, no one has ever seen such a pattern. However, all the other four Yin organs (lungs, spleen, kidneys and heart), often have Yang- or *qi*-deficiency patterns, because of being Yin organs.

Another difference between the liver and the other Yin organs is that the liver has the function of smoothing and regulating the flow of vital energy and blood, which does not conform to *Nei Jing*'s description of a Yin organ's character being to "restore the vital essence but not pour it out". In the Five Elements theory, the liver reflects the character of wood; like trees, its energy grows and moves within its network, and does not like to be suppressed, or stopped, in keeping with the characteristics of Yin. Whereas the the heart, kidney, lungs and spleen can often be seen in a deficient state, the liver is more often seen in a disorder which is not caused by deficiency but by the suppression of its energy.

Gynaecological

Since the liver meridian passes by the genital area, and also has the function of storing the blood, menstruation also relies on the normal functioning of liver energy. Liver-*qi* stagnation can cause PMT, painful periods, prolonged period cycles or scanty bleeding. Even male infertility can be treated by restoring liver energy. Let's have a closer look at the functions of the liver.

Ensures the smooth flow of *qi*

Emotions

The liver function has a deep influence on the emotional state; if the liver-*qi* is flowing normally, the emotional life will be happy. Therefore, some emotional problems can be treated by regulating the liver-*qi*, such as premenstrual tension or premenstrual symptoms (PMT or PMS). The symptoms of mood swings and depression, are caused by tension in the liver (liver-*qi* stagnation) and treatment with herbal medicine or acupuncture to regulate the liver-*qi* can be very effective.

Digestion

In digestion, the smooth flow of the liver-*qi*, not only helps the movement of the stomach- and spleen-*qi*, but also affects the secretion of the gallbladder. Since bile is made from vital liver essence it is important that the liver-*qi* should flow smoothly because if the liver-*qi* is blocked or cannot flow properly, the stomach, spleen and gallbladder will not be able to digest food properly, resulting in indigestion. Apart from the symptoms of tightness in the chest, bloatedness in the abdomen and irritability, which indicate liver-*qi* stagnation, the effects on the stomach can cause flatulence, a sick feeling, even vomiting; and the effects on the spleen cause bloatedness and diarrhoea, etc. The former is called "the liver-*qi* invading the stomach", the latter is called "the disharmony of the liver and the spleen".

Stores blood

In Chinese medicine, the liver is considered as a very important organ for storing blood. It has two functions: it regulates the volume of blood in the body according to physical activity, and it regulates menstruation.

Physical activity

When the body is at rest, or asleep, blood flows back to the liver; when the body is active, the need for blood increases, so the liver will release its storage of blood. In "The Chapter of Formation of the Five Organs" from *Simple Questions* translated by Wang Bing (Tang Dynasty) it says: "Liver stores blood, heart moves it, when the body is active, the blood will move to all the channels; when the body's movements stop, the blood will go back to the liver, that is how the liver stores the blood."

Menstruation

Since the liver stores blood, it has a great influence on menstruation. If the liver stores the blood normally, menstruation will be normal. If the blood in the liver is deficient, the period will be light, even non-existent (amenorrhoea). If liver blood stagnates because of liver-*qi* stagnation, the woman can have very painful periods with blood clots. Or, if there is heat in the blood, this can cause excessive menstrual bleeding.

Controls the sinews and manifests itself in the nails

The sinews (including tendons) are the tissue that holds the bones, muscles and joints together, thus controlling the body's movements. The liver, in turn, controls the sinews because the liver stores the blood, and healthy sinews need to be nourished by blood to enable them to work properly. If the liver blood is deficient, the blood cannot nourish the sinews, resulting in a numb feeling in the limbs, shaking of the hands and feet, difficulty in moving the joints. (In western medicine some of these symptoms could be caused by a stroke, but in Chinese medicine they are considered part of a "liver condition", so the treatment will include tonifying liver blood.

The nails are considered to be the "end of the sinews", so if the nails become dry, cracked, deformed, this will also be attributed to a deficiency of the liver blood, since normal nails need nourishment from the blood. Some skin disorders can also affect the nails. In Chinese medicine, such disorders will be treated with herbs to improve the condition of the liver, and the results can be quite remarkable.

Opens into the eye

The normal function of the eye relies on the nourishment of vital substances from all five Yin organs and six Yang organs, since all the organs are connected with the eye through blood vessels and channels. For instance, the spleen is connected to the eyelid, lungs to the sclera, liver to the pupils, kidneys to the iris, etc. But the liver has the closest relationship with the eye, since liver stores blood, and the liver meridian is connected to the eye, and the eye is the sense organ connected to the liver.

If the liver blood is abundant, the eye will be well nourished, and the vision will be good. A lot of symptoms of the eye can reflect the condition of the liver. For instance, red and itchy eyes, are caused by wind-heat in the liver channel. If the liver blood is deficient, the eye may feel dry, and there may be blurred vision, or night blindness.

In short, the liver is the organ that corresponds to wood in the Five Elements theory; its energy likes to grow and move smoothly. The stagnation of liver-*qi* can cause more emotional problems than the stagnation of any other organs in Chinese medicine. For instance, liver-*qi* stagnation can cause depression, and "liver-fire" can cause an irritable or fiery temperament. Excessive liver-*qi* (or liver-fire) can also invade the stomach and the spleen to cause digestive problems. Since the liver has the function of storing blood, abnormal menstrual bleeding can also be caused by the abnormality of the liver. The eye is the sense organ of the liver, so eye disorders also reflect the condition of the liver. Menstrual disorders and many poor eye conditions can be treated by restoring the liver condition.

The liver and the gallbladder are said to have an interior-exterior relationship: the bile of the gallbladder is formed by the liver and the gallbladder only stores and excretes the bile. Apart from this, the gallbladder is also involved in mental activity, and is said to be in charge of making decisions, or judgements. Pathologically, if the gallbladder is affected by the damp-heat

pathogenic factor, and the function of excreting the bile is affected, it will block the normal flow of liver-*qi*, and cause liver-*qi*
stagnation symptoms and vice versa.

The functions of the spleen and stomach

Of the five Yin organs, the spleen is in the middle, below the
lungs and heart, and above the kidneys and liver. Together with
the stomach, it is the central organ in the production of *qi* (vital
energy). It digests food and absorbs nutrients, sending them to
other parts of the body to keep them well nourished and enable
them to function properly. Although its functions are very different, the spleen is as important as the kidneys. The kidneys
are said to be "the foundation of the innate constitution" while
"the spleen and the stomach provide the material basis of the
acquired constitution". So, "The kidneys are the root before life,
and the spleen is the root after life." The spleen also controls
the blood, keeping it moving along the blood vessels, and the
muscles and the four limbs. It is said that the spleen opens into
the mouth and manifests itself in the lips.

Governs transformation and transportation

If we liken the human body to the government of a country, the
role of the spleen is like that of the ministers of agriculture
and transport who are in charge of the production of food and
transporting it to all the different parts of the country.

In the same way, the spleen digests the food taken in by the
stomach, absorbs the nutrients from the food and transports
them to "nourish the four limbs, the hundreds of bones, the Yin
and Yang organs, the skin and the hair, the flesh and the
sinews". Since the nutrients transformed by the spleen are also
responsible for the formation of the *qi* and the blood, the spleen
is also regarded as "the source of the *qi* and the blood".

If the spleen's food transformation function is strong ("the
spleen *qi* is healthy"), the food can be digested properly, and the
nutrients absorbed and transported properly. If the spleen *qi* is
weak and cannot digest the food properly, the following symptoms may be seen: bloated stomach, poor appetite, loose stool or

diarrhoea, low energy and weight loss. The symptoms of *qi* and blood deficiency may even develop.

Each organ's *qi* flows in a particular direction, and if that direction gets reversed, illness can result. The stomach and lung *qi* flow downwards, upward-flowing lung *qi* would cause asthma and coughs, and upward-flowing stomach *qi* would produce vomiting and nausea. Reversed liver *qi* would cause vomiting of blood, fainting and unconsciousness. One of the characteristics of the spleen *qi* is a "rising" tendency: its *qi* flows upwards to the lungs; if this function is impeded, "sinking" illnesses such as diarrhoea, ptosis of the viscera or prolapse of the uterus may occur. These can be treated by tonifying the spleen *qi*.

Controls blood

The spleen is said to keep the blood in the vessels. If the spleen-*qi* is healthy the blood will circulate normally and stay in the vessels; but if the spleen-*qi* is deficient blood may pass through the vessels resulting in haemorrhages, or ooze out of the vessels causing bleeding. So some bleeding diseases can also be treated by tonifying spleen-*qi*. Uterine bleeding, for instance, can be treated by tonifying the spleen-*qi*, not only because the spleen-*qi* has a "rising" tendency, but also because the spleen-*qi* holds the blood in the vessels.

Governs the muscles and the four limbs

According to *Nei Jing* "the spleen governs the muscles and the flesh of the body". *Nei Jing* also says, "the spleen transforms water and grain into a vital substance (qi and blood), using this to nourish the muscles and the flesh; that is how the spleen governs the flesh (and muscles)." The four limbs also need nourishment from the vital substance which is transported from the spleen. If the spleen is weak, it cannot supply enough *qi* to the limbs, so the muscles of the limbs may become weak and flabby. Therefore, healthy muscles also rely on a healthy spleen function.

Opens into the mouth and manifests itself in the lips

The spleen's process of "transformation" of food starts in the mouth. By tasting and chewing food, the mouth assists the spleen to transform the food. Therefore, the mouth has a functional relationship with the spleen. If the spleen-*qi* is profuse, digestion will be normal, the sense of taste good and the lips moist and rosy. If the spleen-*qi* is weak, there may be lack of appetite, a poor sense of taste, and dry, pale lips. Since the spleen is the source of blood and controls the blood, and the colour and condition of the lips are dependent on nourishment from the blood, the lips may reflect the function of the spleen.

The spleen and stomach are interrelated. The function of the stomach is to receive and store food. In *Nei Jing* the stomach is described as: "the sea of grains and water"; it is like the sea receiving water from the rivers. The stomach, together with the spleen, is known as the "root of the acquired constitution (after birth)"; jointly they digest food, transforming and transporting it around the body.

The functions of the kidneys and the bladder

Kidneys play a much more vital role in Chinese medicine than in western medicine. The kidneys are not only responsible for the metabolism of water and salt, but also for reproduction, growth and development. They are regarded as the "root of life", or the foundation of the innate constitution.

Like the other Yin organs, the kidneys have a Yin and a Yang aspect. The kidney-Yin and kidney-Yang are both equally important to maintain the function of the kidney; they are also the "root" or the foundation of the Yin and Yang for all the other organs. If the Yin-Yang of any other organ becomes out of balance, eventually this will affect the balance of the kidney-Yin and the kidney-Yang and vice versa.

The kidney-Yin is the fundamental substance for birth, growth, and reproduction while the kidney-Yang is the driving force for all the functions that the kidneys perform. The relationship between the kidney-Yin and the kidney-Yang could be likened to a candle and its flame, the candle representing the kidney-Yin and the flame representing the kidney-Yang. The kidney-Yang cannot exist without the kidney-Yin; if the candle is used up, the flame will die out; the kidney-Yin cannot operate without the kidney-Yang, like the candle without a flame. The bigger the candle the brighter the flame. So for the treatment of kidney-Yin- or kidney-Yang-deficient conditions, the remedy of tonifying the kidney-Yin should always contain some substances to tonify the kidney-Yang too, and vice versa.

Although the kidneys are Yin organs and, according to the Five Elements the kidneys belong to water, the kidney-Yang represents fire, and is the source of Yang for any other organ, so the kidneys are regarded as "the residence of water and fire". And no life can exist without water or fire.

Stores essence and governs birth, growth, reproduction and development

The essence of the kidneys forms one of the body's primary substances, and is also the material basis for any physiological function of the body. It is inherited from the parents, and forms the foundation of the general constitution. The essence from the parents (before birth) will also be replenished after birth by the *qi* and the blood extracted from food by the spleen. The kidney-essence has three different forms: the kidney-*qi* (or the vital energy of the kidney), kidney-Yin and kidney-Yang.

The kidney-*qi* is the force that controls growth, sexual maturation, fertility and development. The first chapter of "Simple Questions" in *Nei Jing* describes how the kidney-*qi* controls growth, development, ageing, fertility, and sexual maturation during the various stages of life: it is in seven-year cycles for women and eight-year cycles for men: "for males, at eight years old, the kidney-*qi* is rich, so the teeth will be changed and the hair will grow; in the second eight-year cycle (16 years old), the kidney-*qi* is flourishing, the *Tian-Kuei* arrives, therefore the (kidney) essence is full and overflowing ... in the seventh eight-year cycle (56 years old), the *Tian-Kuei* is used up, the sperm is diminished, the kidney is in decline, both the appearance and the body are extremely (weak); in the eighth eight-year cycle (64 years old), the teeth and the hair fall out." For females, at "seven years old, the kidney-*qi* is rich, the teeth may change and the hair will grow; in the second cycle (14 years old) the *Tian-Kuei* arrives, the Ren channel opens and Chong meridian flourishes so the period comes regularly . . . in the seventh cycle (49 years old) the Ren channel is weak (in energy), the Chong meridian is weak and rear (in energy), the *Tian-Kuei* is used up, the lower channel is blocked, so the appearance is poor, and cannot produce a baby." Both the Chong and Ren channels play an important part in regulating the period. The Chong channel goes up to the head and down to the foot, permeating throughout the whole body and serving as the communication centre for the circulation of *qi*-blood. The Ren meridian, arising from the uterus, is related to conception and is responsible for the supply of blood to the foetus. As both Chong and Ren meridians relate to the period, if the movement of *qi*-blood in Chong and Ren is not smooth, the period will be irregular. The kidney-*qi* is the kidney-essence in its natural and healthy state. The kidney-*qi* determines our basic constitution, strength and sexuality. If the kidney-*qi* (or essence) is insufficient, it not only affects physical and mental development, but it can also be the cause of infertility or impotence.

The hereditary essence and that from food stores in the kidneys, also has another two forms: kidney-Yin and kidney-Yang; two opposite forces within the kidney-essence. If they are in a balanced state, no pathological symptoms will be seen, and the kidney-*qi* will perform its normal functions. If this balance is upset, the pathological changes in the kidney will appear. For instance, kidney-Yin deficiency can cause kidney-Yang "rising", and the following symptoms may appear: a sensation of heat in the chest, palms and soles of the feet, accompanied by night-sweating and seminal emission. Or kidney-Yang deficiency leading to an excess of kidney-Yin can cause fatigue, a cold feeling in both knees and the lower back and an aversion to cold. In men this can result in impotence or premature ejaculation. In women it can result in infertility.

Governs water

According to the Five Elements theory, the kidneys belong to water, so they govern and control the transformation and transportation of body fluids.

The kidneys control water like a floodgate: when it is open, the water runs out; when it is closed, the water stays in. In Chinese medicine, body fluids are transformed and transported not only by the kidneys, but also by the spleen and the lungs. It is said that water is taken in by the stomach, then transformed by the spleen. The pure fluids are transported to the lungs then through Sanjiao to all the organs, and the impure body fluids are transformed into sweat and urine, and excreted out of the body. This process is dependent on the function of the kidney-*qi*: if the kidney-*qi* is weak, it cannot warm up the spleen-*qi* and the lung-*qi*, so their function of controlling water will be weak, as well as the kidney itself. This results in symptoms of oedema and incontinence.

Controls the reception of *qi*

In western medicine, the lungs are supposed to control respiration, but in Chinese medicine, making use of the *qi* (air) from nature, the lungs and the kidneys work together. It is said that "the lungs are in charge of expiration, and the kidneys control inspiration". The kidneys have the function of holding down the *qi* from the lungs, and respiration can only be normal when the kidney-*qi* is strong enough to hold the *qi*. If the kidneys are weak and cannot hold the *qi*, symptoms of shortness of breath and breathing difficulties can appear. This kind of symptom is often seen in asthma cases. So, in Chinese medicine, kidney tonics can often be used effectively to treat asthma.

Produces marrow, fills up the brain, controls the bones

The kidney stores the essence, and the marrow is believed to be derived from this essence. In Chinese medicine, the marrow not only occupies the bone, but is also the substance that "fills up" the brain and the spine. Since the spine connects to the brain anatomically, it is said that the brain is the "sea of the marrow"; the spine and the bone are like rivers leading to the sea.

In *Nei Jing* it says that "the kidney governs the bone" and "kidney produces marrow". If the essence of the kidney is sufficient, the source of the marrow will be rich, so the bones will be well nourished and strong. If the kidney essence is insufficient, the bones will be weak and unhealthy, even under-developed. Therefore, if the closing of a baby's fontanelle is delayed, its kidneys will be weak and fragile. If the kidney is invaded by external pathogens, it may cause insufficiency of essence, so the bones may be "hollow", and cause pain in the back and the knees; the feet may even be too weak to walk. So, the treatment for arthritis with Chinese medicine may include tonifying the kidney.

The teeth are said to be "the end of the bone", so the growth of the teeth also depends on nourishment from the kidney essence. If the kidney essence is weak, the teeth may be weak and loose, and even fall out.

In Chinese medicine, all the emotions, feelings and sensory organs (which in western medicine are part of the function of the brain) are linked up with the internal organs. Chinese medicine didn't include memory until western medicine had influenced China at the end of the last century and the beginning of this century. So, apart from producing marrow the function of the brain has not been well described.

Shows in the hair

It is said that, "The blood and the essence share the same source", since both the blood and the essence receive nutrients from food. The blood is also derived from the essence. If the essence is insufficient, the blood will be weak too. "Hair is the surplus of the blood as it is nourished by the blood", but the growth of the hair is still dependent on the activity of the "kid-ney-*qi*", as *Nei Jing* says: "in a female, at seven years old, the kidney-*qi* is flourishing, therefore the teeth may change and the hair will grow". And, "in a male, at eight years old, the kidney-*qi* is strong, therefore the teeth will change, and the hair may grow". When people are young, their kidney-essence is plentiful, so their hair is shiny and looks healthy; when people are old, their kidney-essence declines, so their hair colour turns to white (according to the Five Elements, black is the colour of the kidney; so if the kidney-essence is strong, its colour should be strong).

Opens in the ears and the two lower orifices

Nei Jing says, "the kidney-*qi* leads to the ears, so if the kidney is in a harmonic state, the ears can distinguish the 'five tunes'." so the ears' listening ability depends on the nourishment of the kidney-essence; if the kidney-essence and the kidney-*qi* are plentiful, the sense of hearing will be sharp. If the kidney-essence is insufficient, the sense of hearing will be weak, and tinnitus may occur. Elderly people often have a poor sense of hearing, because their kidney-essence is in decline.

The external genitalia, external urethral orifice and the anus are functionally related to the kidneys. Because although the excretion of urine is carried out by the bladder, its normal function depends on the activities of the kidney-*qi*. If the kidney-Yang is deficient, symptoms like over-frequency of urination or urinary retention, even urodialysis can be seen. (The relationship between the kidneys and the reproductive system have already been described earlier in this chapter.) Bowel movement is also said to depend on the function of the kidney-*qi*; if the kidney-*qi* is weak, different patterns of constipation may be seen. For instance, either kidney-Yin or kidney-Yang deficiency could be the cause of constipation. If the kidney-Yin is insufficient, it cannot nourish the bowel, so the stool may be dry; and a kidney-Yang deficiency can slow down the movement of the bowels causing constipation. So the treatment for constipation may include tonifying the kidneys.

The kidney channel has an interrelationship with the bladder channel; it is said that the kidney and the bladder have an exterior-interior relationship. The major function of the bladder is to store and excrete urine, but this depends on the "rising" actions of the kidney-*qi*. Pathologically, if the kidney-*qi* is weak, it cannot warm up the bladder, so the opening-closing function of the bladder may fail, then symptoms like incontinence, frequent urination, or difficulty in passing water may occur.

The functions of the lungs and the large intestine

The lungs govern the *qi* (the air and the vital energy), by performing the function of respiration.

Lungs take in fresh *qi* from nature, so, like the skin, they have direct contact with the external *qi*, and act as a screen between the internal and the external environment of the body. So, the lungs are said to be associated with the skin's surface. Another fact that makes the lungs unusual, is that the lungs are Yin organs, but are in a Yang position. They are compared to a *hua gai* (canopy) which, being the uppermost organ, shelters and protects all other internal organs. But the disadvantage of being in this position is that, like the frontier guards, they are more likely to be attacked by the invading army. So the lungs seem to suffer more often than other internal organs. It is said that, "Lungs are delicate organs, vulnerable to the attack of external influences."

Another important function of the lungs is to help to maintain normal water metabolism or "the upper source of water circulation".

The lungs and the large intestine also have an interior-exterior relationship; the lungs have their specific body opening in the nose.

The above characteristics, and the functions of the lungs play an important part in the diagnosis for the treatment and prevention of lungs' disorder. For instance, since the lungs and the skin act as protectors for the other internal organs, remedies such as "Jade Screen" are prescribed, as this contains herbs that tonify the lungs' *qi* and the defending *qi* to prevent colds or flu.

Now, let's have a closer look at the functions of the lungs:

Govern *qi* and respiration

Qi can mean either "vital energy" or the "air" (the cosmic *qi*) that we cannot live without. Both types of *qi* are very important. The lungs' most important function is that of governing the *qi*. They do this in two ways:

Firstly, and most obviously, the lungs breathe in and out the fresh air and used air through the nose, and control respiration. It is said that the pores of the skin also have the ability to regulate "breathing" and to release the *qi*. In *Nei Jing* the pore is called *qi meng* (the gate of *qi*).

Secondly, the lungs govern the whole body's *qi* through the part they play in the formation of the *Zhong-qi* (the gathering *qi*). This is a combination of the food-*qi* (which is transformed by the spleen), and the cosmic *qi* from nature. As it says in *Nei Jing*: "the Zhong-*qi* gathers in the chest, goes out from the throat, fills the heart channel, and controls the respiration." It is also said that "all blood vessels lead to the lungs." So the lungs not only influence the formation of the *Zhong-qi*, but also, through their connection with all the blood vessels, assist the heart to control the blood circulation.

If the lungs' function of controlling the *qi* is good, the breathing will be smooth and even. If the lung-*qi* is weak, or insufficient, it will not only affect the lungs' breathing function, but also the formation of the *Zhong-qi*, producing a group of symptoms that include weak respiration, shortage of breath, low and weak voice, exhaustion, etc. Once the lungs lose their control over respiration, the "fresh" *qi* cannot be taken in and the stale *qi* cannot be breathed out, therefore the *Zhong-qi* cannot be formed, the lungs will lose control over the whole body's *qi*, and eventually the breathing will stop altogether.

Controls the dispersing and nourishment of the skin and hair

The lungs also have the function of dispersing and spreading *Wei-qi* (defensive *qi*) and body fluids to nourish and warm all parts of the body, including the skin and hair. If the lung-*qi* is weak, it cannot nourish the skin and hair, so not only will the skin and hair be dry and look unhealthy; the lungs' dispersing function will also be impaired, so the defensive *qi* will not reach the skin and the body will be easily invaded by exterior pathogenic factors and vulnerable to colds or flu. In Chinese medicine, it is believed that the external pathogenic factors often affect the lungs through the open pores of the skin. When a person catches a cold, the exterior wind-cold obstructs the skin, prevents the spread of defensive-*qi* and interferes with the lungs' dispersing function. A series of symptoms can be seen:

feeling cold (the defensive-*qi* which is part of the Yang-*qi* is blocked and cannot warm the body), feeling hot and sweaty (the body produces more defensive-*qi* to fight the external pathogenic factor), coughing (the lung-*qi* is blocked), and so on. This is how the lungs and the skin are linked.

Controls descending and regulates water passages

The lungs are the highest organs in the body. When the lungs are healthy, the lung-*qi* tends to move downwards, so the person can breathe properly. This is called the descending function. If this function is out of order, the lung-*qi* instead of downwards, will go upwards, causing coughing, wheezing, etc. The lungs' function of descending also affects the water metabolism. The lung-*qi* can guide the water from the upper Jiao (lungs and heart) to the bladder, keeping the water circulation steady. It is said that "the lungs control the movement of the water" and "the lungs are the upper source of the water". Therefore, if the lungs' function of descending goes wrong, the lungs cannot regulate the water or pass it from the upper burner (Jiao) to the bladder, leading to symptoms like coughing up a lot of watery phlegm, a tight feeling in the chest, difficulty in passing water, scanty urination, oedema, etc.

Opens into the nose

The nose is the passage of the air that is breathed in and out by the lungs, so it is considered the "opening of the lungs", and in Five Elements theory, the nose is the corresponding sense organ of the lung. In *Nei Jing*, it says, "The lung-*qi* leads to the nose, and only when the lung-*qi* is in a harmonised state, the nose can distinguish fragrances and offensive odours." This connection can be seen when the lungs are invaded by an exterior pathogenic factor, such as a cold: a blocked nose causes a loss of the sense of smell.

The lungs are connected to the large intestine through their channels. The large intestine has the function of receiving waste from the small intestine and re-absorbing some of the fluids that are left by the small intestine. The large intestine also has the function of excreting stools. It is believed that the normal function of excreting stools is dependent on the descending function of the lung-*qi*. Pathologically, the lungs and the large intestine can affect each other. For instance, in the case of lung-*qi* deficiency, the patient may also suffer from constipation. Since the lungs have the function of governing the *qi* of the entire body, the weakness of the lung-*qi* can weaken the excreting function of the large intestine. This is known as constipation caused by *qi*-deficiency.

The triple burner (Sanjiao) (one of the six Fu organs)

This organ is believed to be one of the six hollow organs, separated into upper, middle and lower portions. Also known as the three body cavities: upper (the area around the heart and lungs), middle (the area around the spleen and stomach) and lower (the area around the kidneys, liver, intestine and bladder). Its function is to regulate the activities of other viscera and participates in the control of metabolism.

The vital substances

Essence, qi, blood, body fluid

If the organs of our body were the mountains of this "invisible scenery", the vital substances: essence, *qi*, blood and body fluids can be likened to the sunshine, streams, breezes, clouds, maybe showers, that give life to and nourish the mountains. There are four different types of vital substances in Chinese medicine, each of which has specific functions.

The concept of *qi* in Chinese medicine

Ancient Chinese believed that everything in the universe was formed by *qi*, which is the most basic substance in the universe. In Chinese medicine, the *qi* refers to two things: the refined vital substances of the body, and the physiological functions of the body. So, one is material, the other is a function; the former is the latter's material basis. This relationship can be likened to that of the candle and the flame. When *qi* flows well, there is harmony and balance, but when it stagnates it is the cause of many illnesses. It is through strengthening *qi* that healing takes place.

There are several different types of *qi*: each *qi* is located in a certain part of the body and performs a different function.

Yuen-qi (original qi)

Original *qi* is transformed from the vital hereditary essence we are born with, and relies on nourishment from food-*qi*. Each of our body's activities depends on the stimulation of original *qi*. Therefore, original *qi* can be regarded as the life force.

Zong-qi (gathering qi)

Gathering *qi* is a combination of cosmic *qi* (air) from the universe breathed in by the lungs, and food-*qi* which is transformed by the spleen from food and drink. These two types of *qi* gather in the chest to nourish the heart and lungs, enhancing and promoting the lungs' function of controlling *qi* and respiration, and the heart's function of governing the blood and blood vessels.

Ying-qi (nourishing qi)

Nourishing *qi* is the *qi* which is transformed from food, and is part of the more refined food-*qi*. It circulates in the blood vessels all over the body, forming part of the blood. Together with the blood, its function is to nourish the internal organs and all other parts of the body.

Wei-qi (defensive qi)

Defensive *qi* is also transformed by food-*qi*, but it flows between the internal organs, muscles and skin of the entire body. It has the functions of protecting the body from attack by exterior pathogenic factors, and of warming and nourishing the skin and the internal organs. It also adjusts the opening and closing of the pores to regulate body temperature.

Blood

In Chinese medicine, the blood is formed by the food-*qi*. As it travels along the blood vessels, it has the function of nourishing the entire body. In *Nei Jing*, it says: "The liver is nourished by the blood, so the eyes can see; the feet are nourished by the blood, so they can walk, the palms are nourished by the blood, so they can hold (things), the fingers are nourished by the blood, so they can pick up (things)." It also says: "If the blood is balanced and functioning well, the mind will be stable." So in Chinese medicine, blood forms not only the material basis for the organs' activity, but also the material basis for the mind.

Body fluids

Body fluids originate from our food and drink. They are transformed by the spleen. They are also dependent on the spleen, lungs and kidneys to transform and transport them around the body. Some of the fluids become sweat, and are transported to the skin by the lungs; some of them are transformed by the kidneys, and are passed out as urine; and many of them are transported by the triple burner (Sanjiao) to all the internal organs to moisten them.

The meridians (*Jing Luo*)

The meridians are linked to the acupuncture needles that play such a mysterious role in Chinese medicine. What are the meridians? And how do they work? *Qi* is said to flow along the lines (or channels) known as meridians and it is these lines that are used by acupuncturists to treat various disorders.

The Chinese for meridian is *Jing Luo*, *Jing* means "road", and *Luo* can be translated as "net". The *Jing* are bigger meridians than the *Luo*. There are two types of *Jing*: the *Zheng Jing* (the regular conduits) and the *Ji Jing* (the odd conduits). Each of the regular meridians connects with a particular internal organ and is named after that organ. There are twelve regular meridians.

The *Luo* meridians, link up these "major roads" forming a

network of meridians covering the entire body, and ensuring a
vital energy flow everywhere.

If this vital energy is blocked or stuck, illness may result. The
locations of the dysfunctions can be either in the meridians or in
the actual organs. Since all the meridians are directly or indirectly linked with the organs, it is said that even if the illness is in
the organs, it can still be treated by regulating the *qi* in the
meridians. For instance, a stomach pain can be treated by stick-
ing a needle in the leg (*Zhu Shan Li*) which is the acupuncture
point on the stomach meridian. Or, for the effective relief of
lower back pain, press the middle point behind the knee which
is the point on the bladder meridian called *Wei Zhong*.

Theoretically, the doctrine of meridian, or the theory of channels and collateral deals with the physiological functions and
pathological changes in the circulatory system and the channels'
relationship with the Zang Fu organs. Most of the pains or
physical changes in limbs, muscles and points are caused by
problems in the meridians, usually blockage of the vital energy.
Therefore, by inserting needles to regulate the vital energy
in the blocked meridians, the aches and pains will disappear.
The meridians and the internal organs are linked both
physiologically and pathologically.

People often confuse the meridians with the nervous system.
They are not the same, although many acupuncture points do
coincide with nerve points. About half of the acupuncture points
are between the muscles, in the tendons and on the skin.
According to modern research, acupuncture affects not only the
nerves but also the central nervous system, the blood vessels,
the metabolism of body fluids and the bioelectricity of our
bodies.

So, a stomach pain is treated from an acupuncture point in
the leg; the message from the leg transfers to the area in the
brain next to the message of pain from the stomach and somehow it affects the feeling in the stomach. Similarly, irregular
menstruation can be treated with acupuncture: the stimulation
message (feeling) from the acupuncture points are sent to the
pituitary gland in the brain that produces the hormone which
stimulates the ovary.

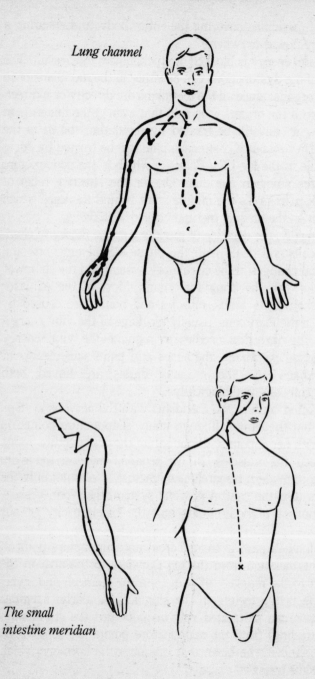

Lung channel

*The small
intestine meridian*

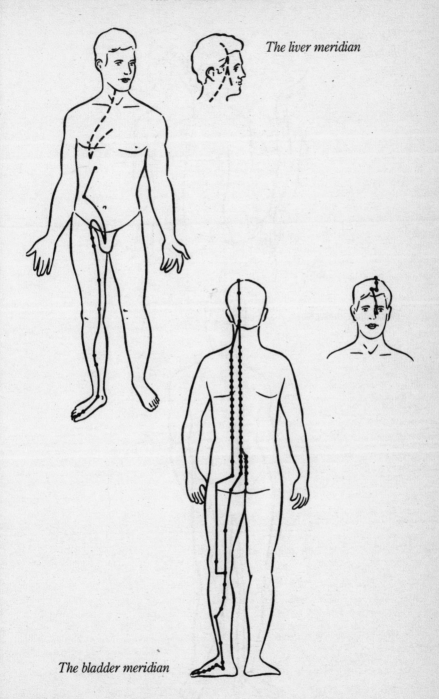

The liver meridian

The bladder meridian

*The triple burner
meridian*

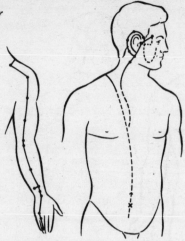

The kidney meridian

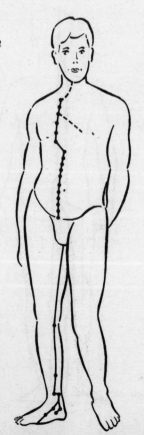

The heart meridian

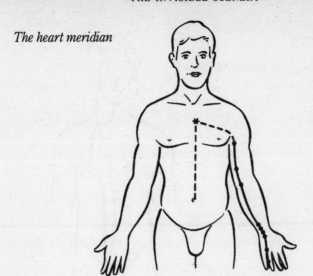

The spleen meridian

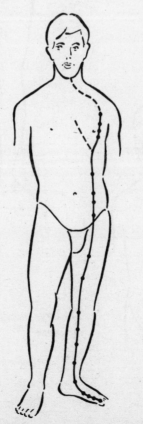

The stomach meridian

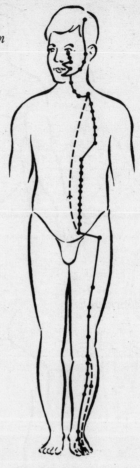

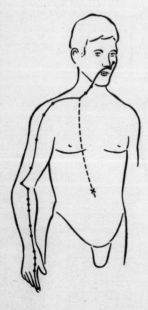

*The large intestine
meridian*

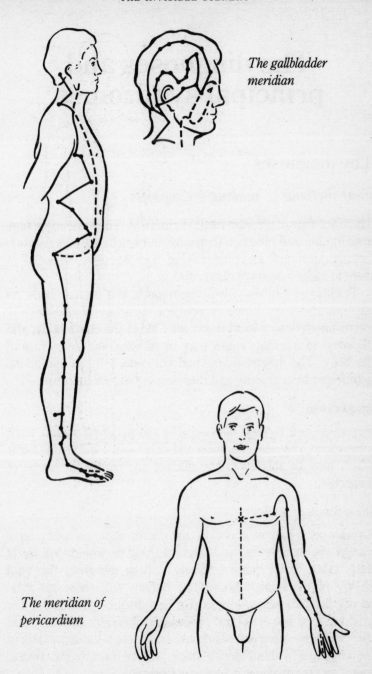

The gallbladder meridian

The meridian of pericardium

5
The diagnoses and principal syndromes

The diagnoses

Four methods of making a diagnosis

There are four diagnostic methods in TCM. They are inspection, auscultation and olfaction (listening and smelling), interrogation (asking questions); and pulse-taking. In most cases, we use all of them to make a sensible diagnosis.

Traditional Chinese Medicine regards the human body as an organic whole, whose component parts are physiologically interconnected, so a local lesion may affect the entire body, and disorders of internal organs may be reflected on the surface of the body. The diagnostic method notes the various symptoms manifested by a disease, and then sets out to find its cause.

Inspection

Inspection is a method of observing the patient's mental state, complexion, physical condition and behaviour – all visible signs which may be related to the disease are within the scope of inspection.

Observation of vitality

As soon as a patient walks in, the doctor should already have started his observation, and the first thing he would look for is the vitality of the patient (*Sheng*). *Sheng* describes the vital energy of the human body. The patient will show his vital energy in two ways: physically (his facial complexion, the brightness of his eyes, and so on) and mentally (thought and consciousness, alertness, sharp responses, etc.). Vitality exists in the physique without which there will be no vitality. Hence, sound vitality dwells in a healthy physique.

Observation of complexion

The colour and lustre of the patient's face are regarded as the outward manifestations of the ability of *qi* (vital energy) and the blood in the internal organs to nourish the body surface. TCM holds that the complexion of a healthy person is shiny and lustrous, and this applies equally to different races.

Physicians in ancient China classified abnormal complexions into five categories: white, yellow, red, blue and black, corresponding to different diseases. A white (pale) complexion is a manifestation of a deficiency of both *qi* and blood; a yellow complexion is frequently related to a spleen disorder and is a manifestation of water retention within the body or deficiency of *qi*. (However, this only applies to yellow-skinned races; white-skinned races would never have a yellow complexion unless suffering from jaundice.) A red complexion generally indicates heat. But there are two types of heat syndrome: excess-heat syndrome and deficiency-heat syndrome. Blue and black complexions normally indicate poor blood circulation but black could also be a sign of a problem with the kidneys.

An experienced physician will always collect as many relevant symptoms as possible, and then put the information together to make the right diagnosis.

Observation of physique

This is to see whether the patient is strong or weak, obese or thin and to find out other facts concerning the torso, limbs and body type. For instance, a strong build indicates sound internal organs and a sufficient amount of *qi* and blood (vital energy), while a slender build indicates fragile internal organs and a deficiency of *qi* and blood. Those of tall and slender build with a deficiency of Yin and an overabundance of fire are known as Yang-organ people. For instance, people who suffer from a chronic cough caused by tuberculosis (TB) or AIDS are usually thin and have excessive fire. While those with insufficient Yang and excessive Yin are usually fat, retaining more phlegm and dampness (a kind of "fat and water retention"). These people are more susceptible to heart attacks or strokes.

Observation of behaviour

Specific behaviour can be an indication of certain diseases so inspecting the patient's posture, gestures, movements, etc. can aid diagnosis. For example, a patient who walks with a slightly bent back might be suffering from lower back ache. A patient who hangs his head, may be short of breath, and reluctant to speak may have insufficient lung-*qi* and kidney-*qi*; a patient sitting with his chin up and having difficulty in breathing with abundant expectoration may have an accumulation of phlegm-dampness in the lungs.

Observation of the hair

Dense black hair is an indication of adequacy of vital essence in the case of Chinese people. If this shiny black hair turns brown, dry and dull, it could indicate a chronic internal organ disorder. Sudden and extensive loss of hair is usually caused by blood-heat with the invasion of wind, and those whose hair thins over a long period of time usually have deficient blood and weak kidneys.

Observation of the eyes

Bright eyes indicate vitality and the person is easily cured when diseased, while lustreless, dull eyes suggest loss of vitality and the person takes longer to be cured when diseased. A yellow tinge is largely due to the retention of damp-heat; red and swollen eyes with burning pain are caused by the wind-heat of the liver channel. Sleeping with eyes half-closed is attributable to a deficiency of the spleen-Yang.

Observation of the tongue

Checking the tongue is a routine part of medical inspection. Any slight change in the body condition will show on the tongue. The tongue, as the sprout of the heart, is related directly or indirectly to all Zang-Fu organs through the meridians, so the vital essence of the Zang-Fu organs can nourish the tongue and any pathological changes in these organs may be reflected on the tongue. Everybody's tongue is different: the colour and texture of the coating (fur), and the colour, size, and shape of the tongue.

Observation of the tongue proper

When inspecting the tongue proper, the physician would look at the colour, shape, size, motion, texture, etc.

The pale tongue

A pale tongue principally indicates cold syndrome and deficiency of both *qi* and blood. It results from the decline of Yang-*qi* leading to insufficient production of Yin-blood or loss of blood by heavy bleeding.

The red tongue

A red tongue indicates heat syndrome and is a manifestation of fullness of collateral vessels with blood surge due to overabundance of heat. A bright red tongue with rough and prickly fur, or thick and yellowish fur suggests excess-heat syndrome, while a red tongue-tip accompanied by red, swollen taste buds indicates a flaring-up of the heart-fire.

The purplish tongue

A purplish tongue can be due to either cold or heat syndromes. The purplish tongue observed in heat syndrome is usually dry because of excess heat and stagnation of *qi* and blood, leading to the consumption of body fluid, while that seen in cold syndrome is usually moist because of the stagnation of blood due to cold which impairs Yang-*qi*, leading to the retention of body fluid.

The enlarged tongue

A swollen tongue which is pale, puffy and tender with moist fur and tooth marks on its margin is usually caused by an insufficiency of spleen-Yang and an accumulation of phlegm-damp.

The emaciated tongue

An emaciated tongue is an indication of deficiency of *qi* and blood, or hyperactivity of fire due to deficiency of Yin.

The fissured tongue

The fissured tongue is a manifestation of a failure of the tongue's surface to be nourished and moistened with Yin-blood.

It suggests three morbid conditions: 1) consumption of Yin-blood due to excessive pathogenic heat 2) inability to supply nourishment due to deficiency of blood and 3) retention of water within the body due to insufficiency of the spleen-*qi*.

The indented tongue

A tongue with tooth marks at its borders is known as indented or teeth-printed tongue and occurs as a result of pressure of the dental coronae on the puffy tongue. So, an indented tongue often coexists with a puffy one. The puffiness of the tongue is due to retention of water within the tongue caused by a dysfunction of the spleen in transporting body fluids.

The prickled tongue

When the tongue's surface is dry and rough, and protrudes like thorns causing a prickly sensation when touched with the finger, the condition is known as a prickled tongue, which is always attributable to an excess of pathogenic heat, no matter where the pathogenic heat is and what stage the disease is in.

Observation of the tongue fur

A normal fur, white in colour and even in distribution, is spread thinly on the surface of the tongue, with its root underneath which is not easy to remove. A morbid tongue fur is caused by an invasion of exogenous pathogens or a retention of phlegm and food inside the body. Inspection of the tongue fur is mainly made by observing its colour, moisture, thickness, appearance and distribution in combination with an observation of the tongue proper.

The white fur

Whitish, thin fur is usually seen in an exterior or a cold syndrome; the normal tongue coating is white and thin as well. In the former case it appears at the onset of an exogenous disease whose pathogens haven't been transferred into the interior of the body with the tongue fur unaffected. For example, the white coating with normal colour may be caused by wind-cold type of cold. Sometimes the white coating also could be seen in the case of sudden onset of internal heat and swift consumption of body fluid, leading to its failure to be transformed in time into yellow because of rapid conversion of the epidemic febrile disease into heat. In this case, the white coating is very dry and rough to the touch.

The yellow fur

Yellow fur results from pathogenic heat, indicating heat syndrome. The extent of yellow coating is related to the degree of heat. So, the deeper the yellow of the tongue coating, the more intense the pathogenic heat. A light yellow, thin fur indicates an invasion by exogenous wind-heat; a thick yellow, dry fur indicates a consumption of body fluid due to internal heat, and is often associated with thirst and constipation; a dark yellow, dry and cracked fur suggests extreme heat.

The grey fur

Grey fur indicates an interior syndrome, which may be cold or heat. In general, grey, dry fur usually occurs in an exogenous febrile disease, marked by fever, and may also be seen in patients with hyperactivity of fire due to deficiency of Yin.

The black fur

Black fur usually appears at the critical stage of an epidemic febrile disease, indicating an interior syndrome, either cold or heat. Black and dry fur, sometimes with a prickle-like coating, is a manifestation of extreme heat and exhaustion of body fluids, often accompanied by such symptoms as high fever, flushed face, a thirst for cold drinks, constipation, etc.

The greasy fur

Greasy fur is a result of a retention of pathogenic dampness and phlegm in the interior and on the tongue due to the depression of Yang-qi, marked by dampness, phlegm, indigestion, damp-heat and so on.

The exfoliative fur

A furless tongue is known as a mirror-like tongue; a tongue with exfoliative fur is known as a map-like tongue; and a scanty and scattered fur on the tongue's surface is called "lingua geographica". In general, exfoliative fur is formed as a result of impairment of both the stomach-qi and stomach Yin, which explains why the exfoliative fur varies in shape. Moreover, the change from the presence of fur to its absence is a manifestation of deficiency of *qi* and Yin and a gradual weakness of vital *qi*. However, the regeneration of a thin, white fur after being exfoliated is regarded as evidence of the conquest of pathogens by vital *qi* and a gradual recovery of the stomach-*qi*.

If the tongue is bright red with a thin, yellow coating, that indicates that there is lots of heat in the body. But a bright red tongue without any coating is a very important sign of Yin deficiency. The former condition should be treated with lots of herbs with a bitter taste to cool the system down. And the latter condition should be treated with tonic herbs, to tonify the Yin. If the latter condition were treated with bitter herbs they would make the deficient condition even worse.

Auscultation and olfaction

Auscultation and olfaction are the diagnostic method of detecting the clinical status of a patient by listening to his voice, his breathing, his coughing, and smelling his bodily odours. According to traditional Chinese medicine, all the sounds and odours from the human body, produced in the course of physiological and pathological activities of Zang-fu organs, may reflect physiological and pathological changes.

Listening to the voice

The voice is produced by the coordinative activities of the larynx, epiglottis, tongue, lips, teeth and nose, and by the functional activities of vital *qi* in particular. Since the lungs control the body's *qi*, the kidneys regulate breathing in and the heart governs speech, the voice is most closely related to those organs.

A loud, sonorous voice often indicates excessive or heat syndrome, while a low, faint voice or disinclination to talk usually denote deficiency or cold syndrome. A low voice accompanied by a stuffy, runny nose and chilliness without sweating are indicative of exogenous wind-cold, etc.

Listening to breathing and coughing

Since the lungs control respiration and the kidneys regulate breathing in, abnormal breathing is mainly related to the lungs and kidneys. A shortage of breath is often due to deficiency of vital *qi* in both the lungs and the kidneys.

Smelling the odours

Foul breath is due to indigestion or a dirty mouth; malodorous belching denotes food stagnancy.

Interrogation

Many symptoms that doctors cannot detect by observation, auscultation, or taking the pulse, can be found out by questioning. For instance, family history; chilliness and fever; night sweating; menstrual cycles; thirst and drinking; frequency of urination and bowel movements, etc.

There are ten questions that should always be asked.

Chilliness and fever

When chilliness and fever occur at the same time, the chilliness is normally considered to be the result of an invasion of pathogens that have a cold nature such as wind-cold. Fever is normally the result of the defending action of Yang-*qi* representing the body's immune system. This happens mostly in the case of influenza or a cold. If the wind-cold pathogens are very strong, and the Yang-*qi* of a patient is very strong as well, the "battle" between them will be more heated, so the patient will go hot and cold. On the other hand, if a patient's Yang-*qi* is very low, instead of having a very high fever with chills, the patient may only have a slight fever and chills so in a way, having a high fever indicates that the body's Yang-*qi* is sufficient, which is not a bad sign.

If a patient has an aversion to cold only and no fever, it could be due to a prolonged insufficiency of Yang or to an invasion of pathogenic cold. This is more likely to occur in a chronic condition or when the internal organs have been invaded by pathogenic cold.

Where there is a fever without any chills, it could be due to an excess of Yang or a deficiency of Yin, caused by an unbalanced Yin-Yang in the internal organs. If a fever occurs intermittently at regular intervals like the rise and fall of a tide, it is called tidal fever. Tidal fever in the afternoon is usually caused by excessive dryness and heat in the stomach and intestine (often accompanied by constipation, a dry mouth and a thirst for cold drinks). Tidal fever in the evening is called night tidal fever and is often due to a Yin deficiency in the lungs or kidneys.

Perspiration

Perspiration is the normal way for a healthy body to release excess heat from inside the body. In TCM, when the body fluid is evaporated by Yang-*qi* it causes perspiration. Normal sweating moistens the skin and its hairs and regulates the nutrient *qi* and defensive *qi*. But some illnesses also cause perspiration when the body is not too hot. Abnormal perspiration wastes the Yang-*qi* and healthy body fluid (a part of Yin), and over a period of time, it will destroy the vital *qi*.

A patient who sweats profusely during the day, even when he does not feel hot, or when he does very light exercise (spontaneous sweating), may be suffering from a deficiency of both *qi* and Yang. In this case, patients often have *qi*-deficient syndromes, such as tiredness, shortage of breath, poor appetite; and Yang-deficient signs, such as an aversion to cold, cold limbs, and frequent watery urination.

Night sweats only happen when patients are asleep, stopping as soon as they wake up. Because this is a bit like a theft (robbers preferring to work in the dark), in Chinese it is also called "theft-sweat". In most of these cases the sweats are due to deficiency of Yin, but some could be caused by both Yin and *qi* deficiency and accompanied by spontaneous sweating.

Aches and pains

Aches and pains are one of the most common clinical complaints. Healthy people should not have any pain. According to TCM theory there are two major causes of pain. Firstly, the blockage of *qi* or blood in a meridian or organ, which we call "the excess type of pain". Secondly, a deficiency of *qi* and blood, so the local organs cannot be nourished which we call "the deficiency type of pain". To find out the causes of pain, the nature, the location, the severity, the frequency, the accompanying symptoms, many questions should be asked, and then a proper diagnosis can be made. Headache, backache, pain in the joints, chest pain, period pain and stomach ache are all very common and in TCM their causes are very different, so questioning is a very important way of making the right diagnoses and giving the correct treatment.

Headaches

This very common condition can be caused by many different pathogens either internal or external.

Headaches caused by external pathogens are usually linked with colds and flu. They are normally acute and accompanied by a sore throat, coughing, runny nose, fever or chills. These symptoms are caused by the blockage of Yang-*qi* (a kind of defensive *qi*) in the Tai-Yang or Yang-Ming channels (both meridians pass the head, one at the front, the other at the back of the head), due to the invasion of wind-cold or wind-heat pathogens.

If a headache always occurs after work, after a long time standing, with tiredness or lack of sleep, it is most likely a deficiency type of headache. This type of pain is usually lingering, moderate, intermittent and long-lasting. So, by looking at the different accompanying symptoms, we can find out which organ's weakness is causing the headache. It could be kidney Yin or Yang deficiency; or resulting from rising liver Yang; or deficiency of *qi* and blood caused by a weak spleen. So, a lot of questions should be asked, such as whether the patient has lower backache; insomnia; dizziness; tinnitus; diarrhoea; or an irritable temperament, etc.

Lumbago

Most cases of chronic pain in the lower back are caused by a kidney deficient condition, since the lower back is the place where the kidneys are located (surprisingly, the kidney channel does not pass that area). Other causes are cold-dampness pathogens, *qi* and blood stagnation, etc.

The lingering pain with a feeling of weakness in the lower back due to kidney deficiency; the pain and feeling of cold and heaviness in the lower back aggravated on cloudy and rainy days caused by an invasion of cold-dampness; and the sharp and fixed pain in the lower back with a limited waist movement all result from blood stagnation.

Pain of extremities

Most cases of pain in the extremities are caused by arthritis. In TCM, the pathogens are wind, cold and dampness. Wandering pain in the joints or muscles (the pain is not always located in one place) is predominantly due to pathogenic wind; static pain with a feeling of heaviness in the affected area is mainly caused by pathogenic cold-dampness; pain with redness, swelling, and a hot feeling in the affected area, sometimes accompanied by fever, is due to heat transformation from dampness. Sometimes patients could have pain located only in the heel, but in most cases, they have lower backache and weak knees as well and it is usually due to kidney deficiency.

Chest pain

Since the chest is the place where the heart and lungs are located, pain in the chest is usually related to these two organs. So, we need to determine whether the pain is caused by a heart problem or a lung problem.

The most common causes of chest pain in TCM are heart-related: deficiency of Yang-*qi* in the chest causing retention of paroxysmal phlegm or stagnation of *qi* and blood leading to obstruction of *qi* and blood in the heart channel; or sudden blockage of the heart channel caused by phlegm or blood.

If chest pain is accompanied by coughing, flushed face, fever, etc., it is probably caused by lung disease. According to the different accompaning symptoms, the causes could be either heat-phlegm in the lungs or a deficiency of lung-Yin.

Hypochondriac pain

If the pain is located in the hypochondriac region, on both sides or only on one side, it is most likely to be caused by liver-*qi* stagnation, or damp-heat in the liver channel. If the former pain always appears just before a period, it could be part of PMT (premenstrual tension) in the case of some female patients, so the treatment should include "moving the liver-*qi*". When the pain is accompanied by jaundice, it is caused either by damp-heat in the liver channel, and/or by gallbladder problems.

Sleeping

Sleep is an indication of Yin-Yang balance in the body. The Yang-*qi* is responsible for making people awake during the day, and the Yin-*qi* is responsible for making people sleep in the night. During illness, the condition of sleeping is abnormal due to uncoordination between Yin and Yang. Deficiency of Yin and hyperactivity of Yang lead to insomnia, whereas deficiency of Yang and overabundance of Yin lead to drowsiness.

Appetite, diet and taste

Since the stomach and spleen perform the function of receiving and digesting food, the appetite and taste are related to them. If a patient feels hungry frequently but can't eat a lot at a time, it means that the stomach's function of receiving food is not working properly. But if a patient has a poor appetite and eats very little, it is probably caused by weakness of the spleen. A sweet taste in the mouth is due to dampness in the spleen or spleen-*qi* deficiency; a bitter taste in the mouth is often due to stomach-fire.

Thirst and drinking

Whether or not a patient feels thirsty; whether he prefers cold drinks or hot drinks are very important signs for judging a patient's body condition. The level of thirst reflects the vicissitudes and distribution of body fluids. Illness without thirst indicates no consumption of body fluids, usually seen in cold-syndrome, while extreme thirst with desire for cold drinks, indicates a consumption of body fluids by excessive heat. A dry mouth with no desire to drink is due to heat in the body caused by a Yin-deficiency condition; thirst that only requires a little bit of cold drink indicates damp-heat.

Defecation and urination

Defecation and urination are two other important signs for measuring the level of heat or cold in the body and the balance of body fluids.

Constipation accompanied by fever and abdominal distending pain is caused by excess-heat in the large intestine. Dry stools accompanied by a red tongue with little fur, and habitual constipation in the elderly, could be caused either by deficiency of Yin or deficiency of *qi*.

Diarrhoea with poor appetite and early morning diarrhoea with abdominal pain are probably due to a deficiency of kidney-Yang. Diarrhoea with an offensive odour and abdominal pain that is relieved after diarrhoea is caused by damp-heat in the large intestine.

Scanty, dark-coloured urine with thirst are attribute to a heat condition; increased urine accompanied by intolerance of cold and a preference for warmth are attributed to a deficiency of Yang or a cold syndrome.

Menstruation

Menstruation patterns reflect the general condition of a woman's health, so asking a female patient about her periods is a very important part of questioning.

Questions about menstruation should include the cycle of the period; the quantity and colour of the bleeding; the associated symptoms; etc.

Periods occurring more than one week earlier at every cycle, often accompanied by heavy bleeding, are known as a preceded menstrual cycle. This is usually due to pathogenic heat or *qi* deficiency. Periods occurring more than one week later at every cycle accompanied by scanty bleeding are known as a delayed menstrual cycle. This is usually caused by a coagulation of pathogenic cold, blood stasis, deficiency of Yang, or blood. Most cases of menorrhagia are due to a deficiency of *qi* and blood, blood stasis, or kidney deficiency. As to its colour, bright red or deep red indicate the heat in blood; light red and thin discharge indicate blood deficiency, Yang or *qi* deficiency; and a dark, brownish, or purplish menstrual flow, with lots of clots is usually caused by blood stasis due to coagulation of cold, and is often accompanied by period pain.

Bad-temper, painful breasts and premenstrual constipation are due to the stagnation of liver-*qi*.

Taking the pulse

Pulse-taking is one of the most important ways of making a TCM diagnosis. It is a very special diagnostic method of TCM. But the skill is very difficult to learn; the only way to learn it is through practice, practice, and more practice. It is not easy for a teacher to describe.

Doctors used to take the pulse more often than we do now. As well as the arteries at the wrists, they used to check the pulses on the head, legs and some other parts of the body. The method of pulse-taking has been simplified since the first book on the subject (*Mai Jig* – the classic book on pulse-taking) was published about 1,600 years ago. The author, D. Wang Shu-He, was the first to recommend the new method of pulse-taking: *Du Qu Cuen Kou* (only check the pulses at the wrists).

Pulse-taking on *Cuen Kou* (wrists) is called: "Three portions and nine pulse-takings". It refers to the three pulse locations on the wrist over the radial artery, namely *Cuen, Guan* and *Chi*, and each pressure-point is felt with light, moderate and heavy pressure respectively to get nine readings of the pulse's condition. This is the most common method of pulse-taking. Each wrist has three pressure-points, so in total there are six pressure-points, each of which may indicate the state of one of the Zang-organs or one of the Fu-organs. So, the three pulses of the left hand can reflect conditions of the heart (the pericardium), the liver (the gallbladder) and the kidneys (especially kidney-Yin), and the lower abdomen respectively, and those of the right hand can reflect conditions of the lungs, the spleen and the stomach, the kidneys (especially kidney-Yang) and the lower abdomen.

The normal pulse

A normal pulse should have three features: *Wei* (stomach-*qi*), *Sheng* (vitality), and *Geng* (root).

The stomach (a Zang-organ) performs the function of receiving and transforming food, while the spleen, its related Fu-organ, is in charge of transporting essential substances. Therefore, it is said that "stomach and spleen are the foundation of the general constitution at birth". So when the pulse is moderate, unhurried, calm and regular, it is said to have stomach-qi. A smooth, even, and forceful pulse indicates vitality. Normally, if you press the pulse hard (near the bone), the pulse will be felt less, whereas if it is pressed with medium force, the feeling of the pulse will be stronger. Therefore, if a forceful pulse can be taken on deep palpation, especially at the location of Chi, it is said to have root.

The abnormal pulse

More than 30 different abnormal pulses are described in modern TCM textbooks, but here are the most common:

Floating pulse

The pulse can only be felt by a light touch and grows faint with pressure. This usually indicates the syndrome which is caused by exterior pathogens, but sometimes it could be found in a deficiency syndrome. It often occurs with the common cold or flu, and in the early stages of some acute febrile diseases.

Deep pulse

Unlike the floating pulse, the deep pulse can hardly be felt by a light touch. This indicates the interior syndrome. A deep and forceful pulse indicates an interior-excess syndrome; while the deep and weak pulse suggests an interior-deficiency syndrome.

Feeble pulse

The pulse is very weak and soft, whether the pressure is light or heavy on Cuen, Guan and Chi. This indicates a deficiency syndrome, and can be seen in both qi and blood deficiency and many other chronic deficiency syndromes.

Replete pulse

The replete pulse, a general term for all vigorous pulses, feels vigorous and forceful at all three locations with both light and hard pressure, indicating an excess syndrome, as seen in cases of excessive heat accumulated internally. This kind of pulse is normally found at the beginning of an illness.

Slow pulse

A slow pulse is a slower rate of pulse beats than normal, usually fewer than sixty beats per minute, indicating a cold syndrome. (In the olden days, doctors would calculate a patient's pulse according to their own breathing speed, so if the pulse was one beat slower than the doctor's breathing, it would be considered a slow pulse.) A slow pulse can be strong or weak, which suggests either excessive syndrome due to an accumulation of cold, or deficient syndrome caused by an insufficiency of Yang-*qi*.

Rapid pulse

A rapid pulse is a faster rate of pulse beats than normal, usually more than 90 beats per minute. This generally suggests heat syndrome; a rapid, strong pulse indicates an excess-heat syndrome; while a rapid, feeble pulse indicates a deficiency-heat syndrome.

Slippery pulse

A slippery pulse is one that comes and goes smoothly, feeling like "beads rolling on a plate", and indicates excess-heat syndrome, phlegm retention or stagnation of food. It can also be seen in the case of pregnant women.

The etiology and the occurrence of disease in Chinese medicine

Chinese medicine divides the causes of illness into three different categories according to the way they affect the human body. This was first mentioned by Chen Yan in his book, *San Yin Ji Yi Bing Fang Luen* written during the Song dynasty.

"Exopathic factors" are the invisible causes which invade the human body from outside, called, collectively, *Liou Ying*. These are natural factors in the form of excessive climatic conditions: wind, cold, summer heat, dampness, dryness and fire.

The mental state has always played an important part in TCM diagnosis. Emotions such as joy, anger, sadness, anxiety, grief, fear and terror, will, when they become excessive, directly damage the internal organs, and eventually lead to physical changes and illness. These excessive emotions are "endopathic factors". They are pathogenic, not natural factors.

Other pathogenic factors such as diet, overwork, injuries caused by falling over, wounds caused by knives or spears and animal or insect bites are "non-endo-exopathic factors".

Exopathic factors

The six different climatic conditions: wind, cold, summer heat, dampness, dryness and fire, would in normal circumstances, do no harm to the human body, However, when they are excessive, or when the human body's resistance is too weak to adapt itself to rapid changes in the weather, these natural factors turn into pathogenic factors. Each different pathogenic factor named after a climatic condition causes a group of specific clinical symptoms. Diagnoses can be made based on these different symptoms.

Wind

The wind, as a natural climatic condition, is regarded as the Yang evil-*qi*; it has an open feature and goes upwards. Sweating is often caused by the invasion of "wind'. The wind pathogen is also characterised by constant movement, and sudden changes, so the symptoms of dizziness, aches and pains moving around the body, sudden strokes, are also caused by the wind pathogen. Since it has Yang characteristics, when the wind pathogen becomes excessive, it tends to attack the upper part of the body; causing headache and dizziness.

Cold

As a pathogenic factor with Yin characteristics, the cold invades the human body in the winter, and with its cold nature, is liable to damage the Yang. For instance, in the case of the common cold or flu, the symptoms of feeling cold and a high fever are due to fighting between the cold pathogen and the defensive-qi. When the defensive-qi is in the winning position, the patient has a high fever, and vice versa. When the cold pathogen invades the internal organs, such as the spleen and the stomach, it impairs their Yang-qi, resulting in abdominal pain and diarrhoea. When the damp-cold pathogenic factor invades the body, it blocks the circulation of the blood and qi in the meridians causing the stagnation of qi and the blood. Symptoms of severe pain in the joints may appear, and warming the affected area with a hot water bottle can help to relieve the pain. Stomach pain or rheumatoid arthritis can be caused by invasion of the damp-cold pathogen.

Summer heat

The summer-heat pathogen attacks the body only in the summer season. As a Yang pathogenic factor, it has hot characteristics and symptoms of high fever, sweating, flushed face, fast pulse, etc. may be seen.

Since the summer heat is a Yang pathogen, when it is excessive, it often suppresses or damages the body's Yin-fluid, and causes a Yin-deficiency condition. Losing Yin-fluid can cause the loss of vital-qi by sweating (through the opening pores). So, as well as a group of heat symptoms and Yin-deficiency symptoms, qi-deficiency symptoms can also be seen, such as fatigue, shortage of breath and poor appetite.

In most parts of China, as summer is a rainy season, the

climate is very humid. Therefore, the summer-heat pathogen often invades the body accompanied by the damp-pathogen. The damp-pathogenic factor causes symptoms such as a heavy feeling in the limbs and a stuffy sensation in the chest (the clear Yang-*qi* is blocked by the damp pathogenic factor, therefore it cannot function and move properly). When the summer heat attacks the spleen and the stomach with dampness, symptoms of diarrhoea, vomiting and nausea can be seen.

Dampness

Dampness not only exists in the summer, but is also common in other seasons. As a pathogenic factor the damp-pathogen has a Yin nature, so it is prone to disturb or damage the Yang-*qi*. Since the spleen is the organ that belongs to the earth in the theory of the Five Elements, it is easily upset by water. If dampness invades the body, the spleen's function of transforming and transporting food and water is affected, resulting in symptoms such as distension of the abdomen, nausea, vomiting, diarrhoea, or water retention in the body, oedema, heavy and swollen limbs, etc.

As a pathogenic factor dampness is characterised by heaviness and turbidity. When dampness invades the body, it often gives rise to such symptoms as a heavy feeling in the head and joints, a sticky tongue coating, or turbid secretions. Arthritis caused by the invasion of the damp-pathogen has the symptoms of fixed pain with a heavy feeling in the limbs and the joints.

Dryness

Dryness as a climatic pathogenic factor invades the body in the autumn, since the autumn is the season that has least rain in most parts of China. Dryness is liable to impair the body's fluid with symptoms of dry and cracked skin, dry tongue, cracked lips, dry stools, etc.

Since the lungs, regarded as the most delicate Zang organs, prefer moist climatic conditions when the dry pathogenic factor invades the body, it would first attack the lungs through the nose and mouth. Symptoms include a dry cough with a dry throat, and sticky phlegm that is difficult to cough up.

Fire

Fire or heat as a pathogenic factor can invade the body in any season, but more often in summer. Unlike the seasonal summer pathogen, the fire pathogen has a Yang nature, with symptoms of high fever, sweating, red tongue with yellow coating, fast pulse, etc. In the case of skin diseases, the skin appears to be bright red, hot and painful. Since fire has a tendency to flare up, it often attacks the upper part of the body, or the Yang part of the body. For instance, the symptom of red eyes (bleeding or inflammation of the cornea) is considered to be caused by "liver-fire"; a red face can also be considered the result of the rising of liver-fire or the liver Yang. A red tongue tip with mouth ulcers is a sign of heart-fire; acute skin infection may be caused by "fire poisoning".

The fire pathogen tends to burn and consume the body's Yin-fluid with symptoms of sweating, thirst, dry mouth and throat, etc. The body not only loses Yin-fluid, but also the *qi* with it. Therefore, apart from the symptoms above, the patient would also complain of tiredness, fatigue, etc.

By exhausting its Yin-fluid the fire pathogen can stir up the "liver-wind" with symptoms of high fever accompanied by coma and deliriousness, etc. Furthermore, the fire may speed up the blood flow causing various types of haemorrhage (when the blood is out of control and flows outside the channels).

The epidemic pathogenic factor

Apart from the above-mentioned climatic factors, the epidemic pathogenic factor is another highly infectious pathogen, which is called *Li Qi* or *Du Qi*. It is spread through the air or by contact and enters the body through the mouth or nose. The onset of epidemic disease is sudden, its development is rapid, and it is often fatal if left untreated.

Endopathic factors

Just as excessive emotions over a prolonged period may eventually cause damage to the internal organs by disturbing the normal flow of the *qi* and blood of the organs, so the imbalance of an organ's *qi* and blood can cause a change in the emotions. For instance, anger injures the liver and affects the smooth flow of the liver-*qi*; joy affects the heart, and excessive joy tends to cause a loss of heart-*qi*; anxiety affects the spleen, excessive anxiety leads to an accumulation of spleen-*qi*, and causes anorexia; fear affects the kidneys and excessive fear can cause loss of control of the kidney-*qi*, leading to incontinence. Sadness affects the lungs, and excessive melancholy leads to a deficiency of lung-*qi*, and causes shortage of breath. The emotions are regarded as the internal causes of the illnesses.

Non-endo-exopathic factors

Improper diet is a non-endo-exopathic factor and includes over-eating, under-eating, or eating fatty and oily foods that are difficult to digest. Insufficient food intake can cause a deficiency of blood and *qi* due to a lack of nutrition. Furthermore, an insufficiency of *qi* and blood could lower the body's resistance, and easily be followed by other disorders. On the other hand, over-eating and an unhealthy diet can harm the spleen-*qi* and the stomach-*qi*, and cause indigestion, vomiting, sickness, bloated abdomen, diarrhoea, etc.

Imbalance between work and rest is another non-endo-exopathic factor. This refers not only to overwork, but also to lack of exercise. Overwork includes both physical and mental work. Physical work can harm the *qi*, exhausting the energy. Mental overwork can cause anxiety and stress, which would eventually damage the heart-blood and spleen-*qi*, causing symptoms of insomnia, poor appetite, etc. Excessive sexual activity is also believed to result in the consumption of the kidney-essence, eventually causing kidney deficiency, with symptoms of weakness and pain in the lower back, vertigo, tinnitus, impotence, etc.

Lack of exercise or too much rest over a long period, may cause retardation of the circulation of *qi* and the blood, with symptoms of poor appetite, weaknes of limbs, excess weight, shortage of breath, etc.

Other non-endo-exopathic factors include traumatic injury

and phlegm retention. Traumatic injury refers to gunshot injuries, burns, knife wounds, insect or animal bites, etc. These can cause bleeding, swelling, fractures, dislocation, and even harm the internal organs, causing the stagnation of *qi* and the blood.

Phlegm retention is a very common pathogenic term in Chinese medicine used to describe some symptoms caused by stasis of water or Yin-fluid in the body. It refers not only to the visible phlegm that we cough up from our lungs, but also to invisible phlegm. Breathing difficulties caused by a heart problem could be caused by phlegm retention in the heart channel. Phlegm retention often refers to water retention in Chinese medicine since they are considered the same condition in a different form. Phlegm retention is regarded as a more condensed form of water retention.

Differential diagnosis and the eight principal syndromes

After collecting information about the causes, a Chinese doctor would then make his diagnosis based on the "Eight Principals", which is one of the most important methods of "differential diagnosis". In Chinese medicine, the diagnosis of illness is based on an overall analysis of the nature and location of the pathogenic factors and the body's resistance. The "eight principal syndromes" are Yin and Yang; interior and exterior; cold and heat; deficiency and excess.

1) *Interior and exterior*
First, we must determine the location of the pathogenic changes and the development of the illness. Illnesses usually start from the surface of the body, and if the body's resistance (the defensive-*qi*) is not strong enough to get rid of the "invader", then it will develop to harm the internal organs.

The exterior syndrome is caused by an attack of any of the six exopathic pathogens through the skin, hair, mouth or nose. It is superficial, mild in nature, sudden in onset and short in duration without affecting the function of the internal organs.

Symptoms include high fever, sweating, sore throat, running and blocked nose.

The interior syndrome is more severe; it signals a pathological change in the internal organs. The interior syndrome may be caused by the six climatic pathogens either superficially or by invasion of the internal organs. Other factors such as emotions and improper diet, also play a part. Symptoms vary depending on the affected organs.

2) Cold and heat

After determining the location of the pathogenic change through the interior and exterior syndromes, the cold and heat syndromes are used to identify the nature of the illness.

The cold syndrome is caused either by the invasion of the cold pathogenic factor, or by a deficiency of Yang and an excess of Yin. Symptoms include an aversion to cold, a preference for hot or warm drinks, a pale complexion, loose stools, clear urine, pale tongue, slow pulse, etc.

The heat syndrome is caused by the invasion of the heat pathogen, or by a deficiency of Yin. Symptoms include fever, thirst, dark and smelly urine, constipation, redder tongue and fast pulse.

3) Deficiency and excess

This determines the body's vital *qi*, and the virulence of the pathogenic factor.

Chronic illness, improper diet, emotional upset, weak general constitution from birth, etc. can all cause the body's resistance (the vital *qi*) to be weak. All these causes may result in various deficiency syndromes, such as blood deficiency, *qi* deficiency, Yin or Yang deficiency, etc. Symptoms include fatigue and weakness, shortage of breath, spontaneous perspiration, weak knees and lower back, pink tongue with little or no fur, feeble or weak pulse.

The excess syndrome refers to the condition whereby both the vital *qi* (the body's resistance) and the pathogenic agent are strong, leading to an intense struggle between them. Symptoms include a strong physical constitution, loud voice, high fever, abdominal distension with constipation, thick and greasy tongue fur, strong and forceful pulse.

4) Yin and Yang

The principle of Yin and Yang is the general guiding principle within the eight principal differential diagnoses, since all the other six principal syndromes can be identified as Yin or Yang syndrome. For instance, exterior, heat and excess syndromes are classified as Yang, and interior, cold and deficiency syndromes are classified as Yin.

It was quoted in *Nei Jing*: "a good doctor first determines the nature of a disease in terms of Yin and Yang by observing the complexion and feeling the pulse." This means that an experienced practitioner would determine his diagnosis first on the principle of Yin and Yang, then more specifically on interior or exterior, deficiency or excess, cold or heat. This diagnosis will guide the treatment, and indicate which herbs to use.

Other syndromes can be used to assist the eight principal syndromes, such as differential diagnoses according to the state of *qi*, blood, and body fluid; differential diagnoses according to the theory of Zang-Fu organs; and differential diagnoses in accordance with the theory of the six meridians.

6

The "sweet and sour" medicine – introduction to herbal medicine

Zhang Zhong Jing (see page 22), said that "[a doctor who] uses herbal medicine is like a soldier using his weapons". Merely having a sound knowledge of the basic theory of TCM will not make a good practitioner. The relationship between the practitioner and herbal medicine is like that of a soldier and his arms. Being familiar with all the herbs and knowing how they work together, and the effect they have on the patient are all-important to the practitioner; just as the soldier needs to know how to use his arms in order to win his battle, otherwise however hard he fights, his chance of winning is very small. So, in addition to a thorough knowledge of the philosophy and the theory of medicine, a practitioner also needs to know the herbs or his chances of healing are very limited. There is a Chinese saying, "Even the cleverest chef cannot make a delicious meal without food."

The theories of Yin-Yang and the Five Elements are not only used to explain the phenomenon of health and illness (physiology and pathology) of the human body, but have also been applied to almost all aspects of TCM. So how do they apply to herbal medicine?

The four properties

If we open a Chinese herbal medicine pharmacopoeia or a textbook of herbal medicine, we will find that all herbs are classified in groups according to their different properties or nature, such as hot or cold, sweet or sour; their meridians and whether they float or sink, etc.

Each herb is ascribed one of the following "properties": hot, cold, warm or cool. According to *Nei Jing*: "To treat a cold condition, hot herbs should be used; and for a hot condition, herbs with a cold nature should be used." This is a fundamental principle of TCM. According to the theory of Traditional Chinese Medicine, it is the imbalance of Yin and Yang in the organs that causes illnesses, so herbs with their hot or cold nature can be used to rebalance the Yin and Yang of the organ accordingly. Basically, herbs with a hot nature have the property of Yang, so are good for a Yang-deficiency condition or a condition with excess Yin which exhibits "cold" symptoms such as an aversion to cold, cold limbs, a pale complexion, very weak pulse, a preference for hot drinks, etc., so herbs with a hot nature can be used to release it, and vice versa. Herbs with a cold nature have the property of Yin, so are good for a Yin deficiency or a condition with excess Yang, which exhibits "hot" symptoms, such as high fever and extreme thirst, a bright red complexion with red eyes, and a fast pulse, all indicating that Yang is predominant. So herbs with a cold nature must be used. In the same way, herbs with a warm property are used to treat a cold condition, and herbs with a cool nature are used to treat a hot condition; their effectiveness is similar to that of herbs with a hot and cold nature, but their intensity is less strong. So, it is extremely important for practitioners to know the properties of each individual herb in order to balance the Yin-Yang of a patient.

The five tastes

The effectiveness of herbs depends not only on their hot or cold properties, but also on their taste. The relationship between the property and the taste of herbs reflects the Yin-Yang philosophy and the Five Elements theory. They complement each other. The five tastes are sweet, sour, bitter, pungent and salty.

"Sweet" herbs are not sharp or harsh, but can be used to

dilute other herbs' toxicity, and make those herbs less harsh. For instance, *Gan Cao* (liquorice) can be described as follows, Taste: sweet; property: neutral; meridian: all twelve channels. So it can be used to tonify the spleen and lungs, to detoxify other herbs, and to reduce the harsh effects of other herbs.

"Sour" herbs are astringent, often used for such conditions as heavy periods, night sweats, or nocturnal emissions.

Most "bitter" herbs have a damp-drying effect, they also have a sinking tendency and very often have a cold nature, so are used for releasing damp-heat conditions such as diarrhoea.

"Pungent" herbs have a moving and dissipating tendency and a hot nature, so are used for conditions caused by blood stagnation, such as headaches, period pain, or any pain caused by injury. Pungent-tasting herbs can also eliminate cold conditions. Ginger, for instance, can be used to treat a common cold caused by wind-cold, or stomach ache due to damp-cold.

"Salty" herbs have a purging and softening effect. For example, *Mang Xiao* (Mirabilite) is commonly used for constipation, *Mu Li* (oyster shell) for scrofula. Both of these have a salty taste.

Meridians (attributive channels)

Apart from its hot and cold property and taste, each herb also has its specific meridians (attributive channels). For instance, *Gan Jiang* (dried ginger) and *Rou Gui* (cinnamon) have a hot nature and pungent taste, but ginger's meridian is the stomach and lungs, while cinnamon only works in the liver and kidney meridian. So, ginger is often used for treating stomach pain caused by "damp-cold" pathogens (symptoms could also be poor appetite, vomiting and watery diarrhoea), while cinnamon is used for treating kidney-Yang deficient conditions, such as oedema, menstrual pain, lumbago, weak knees, etc.

Ascending, descending, floating and sinking

Herbs also have a tendency of action, which refers to the upward and outward effects of herbs or the downward and inward effects.

When a herb is prescribed for a specific condition its tendency of action has to be considered as well as its nature, taste and meridian. For instance, *Chai Hu* (Radix bupleuri), a common herb attributed to the liver channel, is a very effective messenger herb for the condition of liver-*qi* stagnation. Its tendency of action is rising, and, as a famous and effective messenger herb, it can not only lead other herbs to the liver channel to treat the liver condition, but it can also be used to treat "sinking" conditions such as chronic diarrhoea or heavy uterus bleeding because of its upward action. But it should not be used for a condition which has a rising tendency, such as a headache caused by liver-Yang rising, since *Chai Hu* may make the liver Yang rise even more. Another herb, *Niu Qi*, can be used for this kind of headache, even though it is not a well-known herb for the treatment of liver-Yang rising, Since *Niu Qi* has the tendency of sinking, it can be used as a messenger in a prescription to bring the action of the other herbs downward, to treat the liver-Yang rising symptom.

One herb may have several tastes and be attributed to several different meridians. All these considerations must be taken into account, as well as the effect of other herbs. For example:

Fu Ling (Poria cocos)

Fu Ling is a type of mushroom, often found growing underneath the soil near pine trees.

Property: slightly warm
Taste: sweet, almost neutral
Meridians: spleen, heart, lungs, kidneys
Effectiveness: diuretic, spleen tonic; clearing phlegm; relieving anxiety

Clinical use:
1. To tonify spleen-*qi*: to invigorate the functioning of the spleen (and the stomach); to treat oedema and scanty and painful urination.
2. To warm up the spleen Yang-*qi*, stop diarrhoea and reduce swelling. It can also to be used to treat morbid leucorrhoea. *Fu Ling* is very good for treating the kind of diarrhoea caused by spleen deficiency.
3. Clearing phlegm.
4. Calming the *Sheng* or spirit: relieving anxiety or mental uneasiness. It can be used to treat insomnia and palpitation.

Normal daily dosage: 10g–15g.

The composition of the prescription

It is rare in Chinese herbal medicine to prescribe individual substances. When used in a formula, each herb plays a different role. Many formulae are formed by four "ranks" of herbs: *juen* (principal herb), *chen* (associate herb), *zuo* (adjuvant herb) and *shi* (messenger herb).

The principal herb

Juen, the principal herb in TCM, means "emperor", so this one has the greatest effect on the main complaint. It is generally known as the ingredient to treat the cause. In most prescriptions, the dosage of a principal ingredient is bigger than any of the others.

The associate herb

The associate herb, *chen*, means "the minister of the emperor" and it helps the "emperor" in treating the main complaint. Sometimes, the associate herb plays its own role in a formula: apart from treating the main complaint, it deals with some less important symptoms. For instance, if a patient is suffering from migraine and is diagnosed as suffering from kidney-Yin deficiency, the principal herb to be used in the prescription should have the main effect on the kidney-Yin. But if the patient also complains that her migraine always gets worse just before her period and is accompanied by some other premenstrual symptoms, such as depression, irritability, constipation or diarrhoea, the patient has a secondary condition, called liver-*qi* stagnation. So a herb that has the effect of "moving the liver-*qi*" would be prescribed. In this specific prescription, the principal herb should be used to tonify the kidney-Yin, and the associate herbs should be used to move the liver-*qi*. Sometimes, apart from the main complaint, a patient could have more than one less important complaint; therefore, "a few more ministers" can be used.

The adjuvant herb

The adjuvant herb reinforces the effect of the principal or the associate herb; sometimes it can also be used to counteract the side effects of the other herbs in the prescription.

The messenger

The messenger has two functions in the prescription: it focuses the actions of the formula on a certain channel or area of the body; and it can lead the "cure" to the proper meridian, or specific position in the body. For instance, if the pattern of the disharmony of Yin and Yang is only located in the kidney, a messenger herb that has a very strong tendency to the kidney can help the action of the formula to focus on the kidney. The messenger can also be used to harmonise and integrate the actions of the other herbs in the prescription.

These are the principal ways of formulating a prescription. In practice, not all formulae have the four "ranks", but they should all have a principal herb, and one or more associate herbs. If the main ingredients are not toxic, there is no need to use an adjuvant herb.

Classic formulae

The best known book of classic formulae is the *Shang Han Za Bing Luen* (Treatise on Exogenous Febrile Diseases and Internal Diseases) written in 219 A.D. by Zhang Zhong-Jing. It contains 375 formulae, most of which are still being studied as classic formulae in medical schools and still being prescribed frequently by doctors in China.

Patients' conditions can vary so much, that although two patients may have the same principal complaint, the symptoms can vary and if there are coexisting complaints, the formula should be altered. The dosage can also differ according to age and general constitution. Practising the classic formula is very different from studying it, since it is believed that "no two patients' condition is exactly the same", therefore, each patient should be treated individually. So, when studying the classic formula, we must approach it in a therapeutical way: looking at the idea or the spirit within it. Some formulae can contain more than twenty different ingredients, so it is vital to understand what role each herb plays in the formula, i.e. which one is the principal herb, which one the associate, etc.

7

Treating the cause not the symptoms

Clinical demonstration – treatment of eczema

Eczema is one of the most common skin disorders in the UK and China. It is a general term for dermatitis, in which the skin becomes inflamed, appearing red and swollen, even weepy. In Britain the figure is rising every year. According to some reports as many as 15 per cent of children are affected.

One of the causes of eczema is physical: direct contact with certain substances, such as acid or paint. Strong, direct sunshine can also cause inflamed skin. The most familiar cause is biological: bacteria, viruses, fungus, etc. We call it skin infection.

Chronic ezcema cases are more likely to have dry, thick, flaky, rough skin. More adults suffer from this type of eczema. The most common symptom of this type of eczema is itchiness. But most cases of eczema in Britain are caused by allergy. The majority of chronic eczema sufferers in Britain have the condition that is called atopic dermatitis. The term atopic refers to a group of people who inherited the tendency of suffering from asthma, hay fever or eczema. But what are the causes of atopic eczema? The real causes of this allergic tendency are still unknown, but the most common ones are probably pollution, car exhaust fumes, house dust, smoke; and some foods, such as milk, peanuts, eggs, soya beans, bananas and oranges.

To reduce the allergic reaction, this condition should first be treated with steroids and antihistamines. If the skin is infected, antibiotics may also be used. Since the majority of atopic eczema patients suffer from very dry skin moisturising creams and lotions should also be prescribed.

Treatment of eczema with Chinese herbal medicine

According to the theory of Traditional Chinese Medicine, eczema has four different "patterns". It can be caused by dampness, heat, wind, deficiency of spleen-*qi* leading to water retention, deficiency of blood and Yin fluid leading to dry skin. In most eczema cases, there are two or more causes. The causes can be either internal or external pathogens, or a mixture. Dampness and heat are regarded as the most common pathogens to cause eczema. In TCM, one of the important functions of the spleen is to control the transformation, separation and movement of body fluids, so the dampness pathogen could be caused by a weak spleen, especially in the case of child sufferers, who have more delicate spleens. The two most common patterns are damp-heat pattern and wind-heat pattern. I am now going to demonstrate a typical clinical case of a damp-heat pattern of eczema. This may help the reader to understand how the diagnosis of eczema based on an overall analysis of symptoms and signs is made, and how it can be treated with Chinese herbal medicine.

Wet eczema (damp-heat)

Shi Zheng is Chinese for eczema. *Shi* means wet or damp; *Zheng* means rash; most Chinese eczema-sufferers have weepy or watery rashes, which indicate the damp pathogen. The surface of the skin will be broken and become "wet" after scratching, the rashes are normally bright red and, when they have stopped weeping, the rashes will be covered in a yellow crust.

Damp-heat is a group of symptoms which indicate not only a special type of weeping eczema, but also the patient's body condition. The dampness can easily be identified by the wet skin rash, while the bright red-coloured rash indicates heat. At the same time, the pulse, the tongue and many other symptoms, such as an aversion to heat and preference for cold drinks, constipation and sweating, also indicate heat.

The treatment should include clearing the heat and the dampness. For patients who have a weak spleen, such as children or those who suffer from diarrhoea, some herbs for tonifying the spleen should be prescribed. The herbs listed below are commonly used to treat this type of eczema.

Chang Zhu (Rhizoma pinelliae)
Huang Bai (Cordiex phellodendri)
Ku Sheng (Sophora flavescens), "bitter root"
Dan Zhu Ye (Herbra lophatheri)
Sheng Di Huang (Radix rehmanniae)
Hua Shi Fen (Talcum)
Sheng Gan Cao (Radix glycyrrhizae)
Yi Yi Ren (Semen coicis)
Fu Ling (Poria cocos), Hoelen
Bai Zhu (Atractylodes macrocephalae) Atractylodes
Bai Xian Pi (Dictamnus dasycarpus)
Di Fu Zi (Fructus kochiae)

A typical formula includes:

Er Miao San ("two magical herbs" . . . *Huang Bai* and *Chang Zhu*)

Case History

David, a thin boy, aged five with dry hair and an irritable temperament. First visited the clinic in March 1993. His mother gave these details:

History: Grandfather had asthma. David started suffering from eczema at three months. The condition gradually got worse over the years. In the last six months, he had been getting one skin infection after another, having been prescribed various antibiotics and topical steroids. But the condition had not been handled well and he had to be hospitalised for a week.

Complaint: Severe itchiness all over the body, constant scratching, the skin lesions caused by scratching are weeping and bleeding. Disturbed sleep, poor appetite, raging thirst, drinks lots of fluid and prefers cold drinks. Likes sweet foods but doesn't eat proper meals. Opens bowels 2–3 times a day, loose stool.

Examination: Eczema all over the body, bright red rashes covered with yellowish crust on the face; red patches with flaky skin on arms and legs; ankles covered with spotty rashes, fingers swollen, reddish like carrots and partly cracked.

Tongue: Thick and sticky at the back, slightly yellow and thin coating at the tip of the tongue with bright red property.

Pulse: Slippery and fast, but spleen pulse weak.

Treatment

FIRST VISIT: This is a typical case of "wet" eczema, caused by a damp-heat pathogenic factor. According to the TCM diagnoses, his spleen-*qi* is weak, having been attacked by the wind-heat external pathogen. Since the spleen is weak, its function of transporting the body fluids is weakened, so the body fluids are stagnant, forming the internal pathogenic factor, the dampness. If the dampness can't be cleared for a long period of time, it will stop the heat being released from the body and will form the internal pathogen of damp-heat. The damp-heat pathogen could also be formed in a patient who has a Yin-deficient general constitution (called "empty heat" or a lack of cold property in the body) as well as a weak spleen or a spleen invaded by the external pathogen of dampness.

David's skin lesion, tongue and pulse all indicated dampness and heat, so the principle of the treatment had to be "clearing the dampness and the heat". Since this patient had signs of a weak spleen, and children's organs are considered very delicate anyway, especially their digestive systems, the prescription for this particular patient should exclude those with a very cold nature and bitter taste, since they would upset the spleen and stomach. Proper treatment should include herbs to tonify the spleen and clear the damp-heat.

The spleen also has the function of transforming the food and transporting the nutrients to the lungs to form the *Wei-qi* (defensive-*qi*). If the spleen is functioning properly, the defensive-*qi* will be strong, and the external pathogens (such as bacteria) will have no chance to invade the healthy body. So, by tonifying the spleen, the external "wind-heat" pathogens, which would make the skin red and itchy, can be kept at bay.

The following prescription was given:

Bai Zhu (Atractylodes macrocephala) 9gm, *Fu Ling* (Poria cocos) 6gm, *Chen Pi* (Citrus reticulata) 6gm, *Huang Qin* (Radix scutellariae) 9gm, *Shen Di Huang* (Radix rehmanniae) 6gm, *Shen Gan Cao* (Radix glycyrrhizae) 6gm, *Hua Shi* (Talcum) 9gm, *Dan Zhu Ye* (Herbra lophatheri) 9gm, *Jing Jie* (Herbra schizonepetae) 9gm, *Fang Feng* (Radix ledebouriellae) 9gm, *Bai Xian Pi* (Cortex dictammiradicis) 9gm.

The principal herb
Huang Qin was prescribed to clear the dampness and the heat so as to reduce the weepiness and redness of the skin.

The associate herbs
Bai Xian Pi, Jing Jie and *Fang Feng* were prescribed to clear the wind-heat and to stop the itchiness.
Bai Zhu, Fu Ling and *Chen Pi* were prescribed to tonify the spleen so as to reduce the dampness and improve the digestion.
Shen Di Huang was prescribed to assist the *Huang Qin* to clear the heat.

Adjuvant herbs
Hua Shi and *Dan Zhu Ye* were prescribed to lead the heat out of the body through the urine.
Sheng Gan Cao was prescribed to clear the heat, as well as to neutralise the harshness of the herbs with a cold nature, and to reduce the bitter taste with its sweet taste.

SECOND VISIT: David's mother said that the itchiness was less severe so he was scratching less; he was sleeping better, but the skin lesions were still slightly weepy, and the stool still slightly loose. The bowel movement was also frequent. The tongue and the pulse were slightly better than the last time.

Treatment

The principle of the treatment was the same, but fewer herbs were needed to clear the heat and some more were needed to tonify the spleen.

Prescription:

Bai Zhu 9gm, *Fu Ling* 9gm, *Chen Pi* 6gm, *Shang Yao* (dioscorea opposita) 9gm, *Cang Zhu* (atractylodes lancea) 9gm, *Huang Qin* 6gm, *Shen Di Huang* 6gm, *Shen Gan Cao* 6gm, *Hua Shi* 9gm, *Dan Zhu Ye* 9gm, *Jing Jie* 9gm, *Fang Feng* 9gm.

THIRD VISIT: The boy is much more cheerful. His mother said: "David's skin has now stopped weeping, and the skin all over the body is softer, although he still has some pinkish patches on the back of his knees and both ankles. He now sleeps very well at night, his appetite has increased, and he only scratches when he gets upset."

Treatment

Since the weepiness has stopped, indicating that the dampness is much less, and the spleen is better than before, the signs of wind-heat are also less. Therefore, the treatment will concentrate on clearing the heat in the blood, and tonifying the spleen to prevent the eczema returning.

Prescription

Bai Zhu 9gm, *Chen Pi* 6gm, *Shang Yao* 9gm, *Mu Dan Pi* 6gm, *Shen Di Huang* 6gm, *Shen Gan Cao* 6gm, *Hua Shi* 9gm, *Dan Zhu Ye* 9gm, *Fang Feng* 9gm.

Conclusion

For patients who suffer from damp-heat eczema, the treatment normally starts with clearing the heat and the dampness. The damp-heat pathogen, often combined with the wind, can cause terrible itchiness. The heat often stays not only skin deep, but in the blood, so herbs which can clear the heat in the blood should also be used. Since children's spleens are more easily upset by medicines with a cold nature, tonifying the spleen should also be considered throughout the course of treatment, since the spleen is also the organ responsible for transporting the body fluids, so by treating the spleen, you can also reduce the dampness as well as preventing a recurrence of the eczema.

The treatment for this type of eczema can take up to a few

weeks to clear the damp-heat pathogen, depending on the individual patient. Once the damp-heat is gone, and the skin is not weepy any more, the rest of the treatment will be easier but will take longer, and will involve herbs to tonify the spleen and the blood, and to clear the heat from the blood. The dosage will be reduced until it is completely cleared, leaving the skin nice and smooth.

8

Living for ever: food therapy, Tai Chi and Qi Gong

Food therapy and tonic herbs

TCM emphasises the prevention of disease, before and during treatment. That is why over several thousands of years we have discovered so many tonic herbs, such as *Ginseng*, *Ling Zhi* and hundreds of others.

Traditional Chinese medicine could also be regarded as an art of maintaining well being. People learn about TCM, not necessarily just for the purpose of being a doctor, but for the sake of their own fitness, health, and long life, in which diet plays an important part.

"Medicine and food have the same source" is a Chinese saying. Sheng Nong (see page 24) not only taught people how to identify herbs, but also how to raise crops. The character of the word "medicine" in Chinese used to be written with the lower part of the picture as an ancient wine pot.

Rice wine is considered a special food or medicine which has a very hot nature. It can be used to help blood circulation and to release the pain caused by blood stagnation in, for instance, bruises caused by injury. Our forefathers realised that wine was such a special food that not only could it be used as a medicine on its own, but by mixing it with other foods or herbs, it could make lots of other useful medicines. The most common form of Chinese herbal medicine was probably tincture. That is the most likely explanation for the picture of the wine pot in the lower part of the character of the word "medicine".

Apart from Chinese rice wine, many other foods can be used as medicines. Spring onions and ginger are used for colds caused by the "wind-cold" type of external pathogens; sesame seeds are used as a medicine for tonifying Yin and the blood, and are also good for constipation; peanut skins are supposed to stop bleeding; but the walnut is for tonifying kidney-Yang . . . .

Herbal medicines can make delicious foods as well. For example, *Fu Ling* is a herbal medicine that can be used for treating diarrhoea, poor appetite and insomnia. Mixed with sugar and rice flour, it can be made into a cake. *Fu Ling* cake was a famous court food in the Qing dynasty, and can still be found in food shops in Beijing.

Although the leaves of *Gou Qi Zi* have a bitter taste, if you stir fry the fresh leaves, it makes a very delicious dish that is good for high blood pressure and blurred vision. Lotus leaves have the effect of clearing summer heat and damp and can be used to make a sticky rice cake known as Dim-Sim, a wonderful food with an exotic smell of fresh leaves.

Foods and their medicinal properties

Vegetables

Name	Nature & Taste	Meridian	Effect	Clinical use
GINGER	Warm, spicy	Stomach, spleen, lungs	Dispels wind-heat, warms the stomach meridian and stops vomiting, detoxifies	Common colds caused by wind-heat; vomiting caused by food poisoning from fish or shellfish
SPRING ONION	Warm, spicy	Stomach, lungs	Dispels wind-heat, warms the Yang-*qi*	Common colds caused by wind-heat, diarrhoea with pain in the stomach, scanty urination caused by deficiency of Yang

Name	Nature & Taste	Meridian	Effect	Clinical use
CORIANDER	Warm, slightly pungent	Stomach	Moves the stomach-*qi* downwards	Indigestion
POTATO	Warm, sweet	Stomach, spleen	Tonifies the stomach and spleen	Stomach or duodenal ulcer, constipation
PEPPER-MINT	Cold, spicy	Lungs, liver	Clears wind-heat, soothes the throat and moves the liver-*qi*	Colds caused by wind-heat, sore throats, blocked nose, period pain caused by liver-*qi* stagnation, PMT
SPINACH	Neutral	Large intestine, liver	Tonifies blood, stops bleeding	Tooth bleeding, constipation, anaemia
CABBAGE	Warm, neutral	Stomach, spleen		Stomach and duodenal ulcer, poor appetite
CUCUMBER	Cold sweet	Stomach, kidneys	Clears heat poison and damp-heat	Oedema, cold sores
POTATO	Slightly cold, sweet, sour	Stomach, liver	Clears heat in the stomach, and improves appetite	Gum bleeding, poor appetite
GARLIC	Warm, spicy	Stomach, large intestine	Treats TB, prevents flu, stops diarrhoea	Diarrhoea, flus or colds, coughs caused by TB
CELERY	Cool	Liver	Clears heat and dampness, reduces the liver-Yang rising	Irregular periods, heavy bleeding, headaches caused by liver-Yang rising

Name	Nature & Taste	Meridian	Effect	Clinical use
TURNIP	Cool, sweet	Lungs, spleen	Clears phlegm and stops coughing, moves the *qi* in the stomach and spleen	Coughs with a lot of mucus, feeling full and bloated in the stomach
CARROT	Warm	Liver, spleen	Tonifies spleen and liver	Indigestion, dry eyes, blurred vision, especially at night

Fruits

Name	Nature & Taste	Meridian	Effect	Clinical use
APPLE	Cool, sweet, sour	Large intestine, spleen	Tonifies spleen, clears heat	Thirst, diarrhoea
PEAR	Cool, sweet, sour	Lungs, stomach	Tonifies lung-Yin and stops coughing, clears heat in the stomach	Coughs caused by wind-heat, thirst caused by heat in the stomach
BANANA	Cold, sweet	Large intestine, lungs	Clears heat and nourishes the large intestine	Constipation, dry coughs
DATES	Warm, sweet	Spleen, stomach	Tonifies spleen and *qi*, nourishes blood and calms the *Shen*	Fatigue caused by deficiency of *qi*
WATER MELON	cool, sweet	heart, stomach, bladder	Clears heat, reduces water retention	Hotness and irritability, oedema

Name	Nature & Taste	Meridian	Effect	Clinical use
LOTUS ROOT	Cool, sweet	Liver, heart, spleen, stomach	Clears heat and stops bleeding, and moves the blood	Vomiting blood or coughing with blood, heavy periods
GRAPE	Warm, sweet, sour	Spleen, kidneys	Tonifies *qi* and the blood, reduces water retention, calms the foetus	Weakness, morning sickness, oedema
OLIVE	Neutral, sweet, sour	Stomach, lungs	Clears heat-poison, promotes secretion of body fluids (saliva)	Sore throat, dry mouth
KIWI FRUIT	Cool, sweet, sour	Kidneys, liver	Clears damp-heat in kidneys and liver	Kidney stones, jaundice
LYCHEE	Warm, sweet, sour	Liver, spleen, kidneys	Tonifies liver, spleen, and kidney essence	Coughs with *qi*-deficiency, shortage of breath, chronic diarrhoea
HAWTHORN BERRY	Warm, sweet, sour	Stomach, spleen, liver	Tonifies spleen, and helps digestion; moves the blood and stops pain	Indigestion (especially after big fatty meal), period pain, high cholesterol and blood pressure
WATER CHESTNUT	Cold, sweet	Lungs, stomach	Reduces blood pressure	High blood pressure
ORANGE	Warm, sweet and sour	Lungs, stomach	Helps digestion, removes wind in the spleen and stomach	Indigestion, bloated stomach, and too much wind

Nuts

Name	Nature & Taste	Meridian	Effect	Clinical use
WALNUT	Hot, sweet	Kidneys, large intestine	Tonifies the kidney-Yang and nourishes the large intestine	Constipation, lower back pain, impotence
ALMOND	Cool, bitter	Lungs, large intestine	Clears phlegm and stops coughing, soothing the large intestine	Coughs with phlegm, constipation
PEANUT	Neutral, slightly sweet	Spleen, lungs	Tonifies the spleen and reduces oedema, increases the secretion of milk	Oedema, not enough milk after labour
CHESTNUT	Warm, sweet	Kidneys, spleen	Tonifies the kidneys and spleen-Yang	Back pain, diarrhoea
PINE NUT	Cool, sweet	Lungs, large intestine	Stops coughing	Coughs, constipation
PEACH KERNEL	Warm, sweet, bitter	Heart, liver, large intestine	Moves stagnant blood, nourishes the large intestine	Constipation, period pain with many blood clots, pain caused by appendicitis, coughs with chest pain and yellow phlegm

Flowers

Name	Nature & Taste	Meridian	Effect	Clinical use
JASMINE	Cool	Liver, spleen, stomach	Moves liver-*qi*, tonifies the spleen and stomach	Poor appetite, bloated stomach, stomach pain or period pain
ROSE	Warm, sweet	Liver	Moves blood and *qi*, regulates periods	Period pain, irregular periods
CAMOMILE	Cool, sweet	Liver, lungs	Clears wind-heat and liver-fire	Headaches caused by liver-Yang and red eyes by wind-heat
HONEY-SUCKLE	Cool, bitter	Lungs	Clears heat and fire poisons	Acne, coughs with yellow phlegm, sore throat

Meat

Name	Nature & Taste	Meridian	Effect	Clinical use
CHICKEN	Warm, sweet	Spleen, stomach	Tonifies *qi* and the blood	Weakness after giving birth and illness
BEEF	Warm, sweet	Liver, kidneys	Tonifies the blood	Anaemia, kidney deficiency
PORK	Neutral, sweet, salty	Spleen, stomach, kidneys	Tonifies *qi* and Yin	After labour or illness as a tonic food
LAMB	Warm	Kidneys, lungs	Tonifies kidney-Yang	Feeling cold, pain in lower abdomen during period

Fish

Name	Nature & Taste	Meridian	Effect	Clinical use
PRAWN	Warm, sweet	Kidneys, liver	Increases secretion of milk, tonifies kidney-Yang	Secreting little milk after labour, impotence
MUSSEL	warm, salty	Kidneys, liver	Strengthens liver and kidneys, tonifies the blood and essence	Weakness caused by chronic illness, impotence
CARP	Neutral, sweet	Spleen, stomach, large intestine	Reduces oedema, increases secretion of milk	Oedema, a shortage of milk after labour

Other foods

Name	Nature & Taste	Meridian	Effect	Clinical use
VINEGAR	Warm, sour, bitter	Liver, stomach	Releases pain from intestinal ascariasis; softens fish bone	Severe stomach pains caused by intestinal ascariasis; fish bone stuck in throat
HONEY	Sweet	Spleen, lungs	Tonifies the *qi*	Poor appetite, insomnia
SESAME OIL	Cool, sweet	Large intestine	Nourishes the large intestine	Constipation
CINNAMON	Hot, sweet, spicy	Kidneys, liver, heart, spleen	Warms up the middle Jiao, tonifies kidney-Yang, warms the meridians and moves *qi* and blood	Stomach pains, impotence and frequent urination, diarrhoea, period pain, arthritis
TEA	Cool, bitter, sweet	Heart, lungs, stomach	Stops diarrhoea, clears heat, detoxifies	Diarrhoea, detoxifies poisoning by gas
RICE	Neutral, sweet	Spleen, stomach	Tonifies spleen-*qi* and soothes the stomach	Diarrhoea, poor appetite
COW'S MILK	Neutral, sweet	Lungs, stomach	Tonifies *qi* and blood, nourishes the stomach and detoxifies	Weak general health caused by chronic illness, detoxifying poisoning by mercury and arsenic
GOAT'S MILK	Warm, sweet	Spleen, kidneys	Tonifies *qi* and the blood	Chronic illness, poor appetite

Treatment of common illnesses with food

PMT, PMS

Premenstrual tension or premenstrual sydrome is a very common condition in female patients. According to traditional Chinese medicine, there are a few different clinical types of PMT which are caused by disorders of different internal organs. The most common types are liver-*qi* stagnation and deficiency of spleen-*qi*.

Liver-*qi* stagnation

If a patient always feels depressed or tearful before her period (whether or not her stomach is bloated), it indicates stagnation of liver-*qi*. Since the liver has the function of storing blood and controlling the movement of *qi*, it is closely related to the emotions. Therefore, the treatment should be to move the liver-*qi*.

Prescription:

Using one tea bag of peppermint tea make a mugful of tea. Drink two or three cups a day, starting 7–10 days before the period starts properly.

Deficiency of spleen-*qi*

If the patient has a loose bowel or diarrhoea a few days before her period and slight oedema, and feels tired, she may have a deficiency of spleen-*qi*.

Prescription:

Mix 2–3 teaspoons of honey with warm water and drink this every night before going to sleep.

Eczema

Eczema is a condition related to heat and dampness; the wind is normally an external pathogen, caused by food. Therefore the treatment should also include the avoidance of certain foods.

Foods which can make eczema worse include: shellfish, milk products (especially cheese), chocolate, oranges, spicy foods, deep-fried foods, very salty food, etc.

Some foods can clear heat or dampness, and are good for eczema: cucumber, celery, pears, water melon, water chestnut, mint, camomile, etc.

Here is a typical recipe:

Cook 50–100gm of fresh honeysuckle flower with one pint of cold water for 20 minutes, then add two peppermint tea bags. Cook for another five minutes. Wait until it cools down a bit, then strain the herbs. To the liquid add 2 teaspoons of honey, stir well, divide it into two portions. Drink one portion in the morning and one in the evening. If necessary, repeat the next day. Avoid the foods listed above.

Constipation

Eat 1–2 bananas in the morning before breakfast. Or take 15-30 mls of sesame oil twice a day.

Coughs

In Chinese medicine, coughs are divided into many different types according to their causes. They are considered to be caused by the wind. According to different symptoms, coughs are wind-heat or wind-cold.

Wind-heat coughs

These are dry with a headache, fever, severe thirst or dry mouth, constipation, etc.

Recipe: Cook 18gm camomile flowers or 2 camomile tea bags with 9gm peeled almond kernels in a pint of water for half an hour. Strain. Drink it cold, twice a day.

Wind-cold coughs

Symptoms are: cough with a headache, stiff neck, white phlegm, shivers, feeling cold, etc.

Recipe: Peel and chop one white turnip and one pear, then

add seven white peppercorns and 50gm honey. Put all the ingredients in a large bowl and set inside a saucepan containing some cold water. Steam for 30 minutes.

Common cold

Wind-cold

Recipe: Finely chop 10gm fresh ginger (about 3–5 slices). Put it in a mug and add boiling water. Cover and leave for 5 minutes. Then stir in 1–2 teaspoons of brown sugar. Drink it hot, so it makes you sweat.

Wind-heat

Recipe: Put 6gm chrysanthemum or 1 tea bag and 6gm peppermint or 1 tea bag together in a mug. Add boiling water. Leave for 5 minutes, then add 1 teaspoon honey. Drink it twice a day.

Period pain

In Chinese medicine, the cause of pain is usually the blockage of blood or *qi*. Either the hot or the cold pathogenic factor can cause the blockage, but the cold is more common. If it is caused by the cold, the patient should avoid eating very cold food, like ice-cream, freezing cold drinks, etc.

Recipe: Soak 450gm walnuts, 225gm sugar, 12gm pepper in rice wine for 10 days. Then eat three soaked walnuts a day.

If the period pain is caused by heat avoid hot and spicy food.

Recipe: Add 30gm hawthornberry and 9gm peach kernel to one pint of water and cook for half an hour. Drink twice a day for five days, starting seven days before the period.

Acne

According to Chinese medicine acne is caused by heat, or "fire-poison". Therefore the treatment will include clearing the heat and the fire.

Some foods will increase the heat: chocolate, cheese, full fat milk, butter, very oily food, citrus fruit, spicy food, wine, etc.

Recipe: Eat plenty of cucumber and carrot salads; also pears and water melon, and use rice vinegar externally on the acne, several times a day.

Cystitis

Cystitis is caused by infection, or, in Chinese medicine, by "damp-heat" in the bladder meridian. The patient should drink plenty of water in order to clear the heat through the urine. The patient should also avoid all hot and spicy foods.

Recipe: Chop 2kg celery and steam it to make a liquid. Drink 2–3 cups a day. Water melon, pears, lotus root, water chestnuts are also good for this condition, so eat plenty of them.

Qi Gong *and* Tai Chi

We have seen how food can alter our health and balance the Yin and Yang in our bodies. *Qi Gong* and *Tai Chi* is also a good way of improving our health and fitness. Also part of TCM they are based on the same principle of Yin and Yang and the theory of meridians which allow the vital energy to flow. There are many types of *Qi Gong; Tai Chi* could be considered as one of them, although it contains more physical movement than mental concentration or meditation. Everyone who has been to China must have seen people practising *Qi Gong* or *Tai Chi* in the park in the early morning with slow and gentle body movements.

Chinese massage (*Tuei Na*) is more like osteopathy, used mainly for chronic pain or acute muscle or bone injury. It is a kind of treatment using manipulation by hands, not medicine or needles. It is not used for depression or stress relief. But for a baby, massaging certain points on a special meridian, can treat many internal organs' disorders. Now it is starting to be separated from the traditional relaxation massage. Named as "Baby Tuei Na".

For most westerners, acupuncture is the most familiar part of TCM. Also based on the Yin-Yang philosophy and the Five

Elements theory, the treatment aims directly at the points on a meridian with very thin needles. We believe that every meridian is linked to a certain organ, so if the Yin-Yang balance of an organ is not right, it will be reflected in certain points on its channel. By stimulating certain points on the channel, you can also alter the troublesome organs. Why it works and how it works is not the purpose of this book, but if you are interested in it, there are many book available on the subject.

9

Practical questions and answers about herbal medicine

General questions

What is Chinese herbal tea?

A lot of people refer to Chinese herbal medicine as "Chinese herbal tea". I don't know why it is called herbal "tea"; in fact, its taste is nothing like tea, it's actually probably closer to a sort of concentrated coffee, but with a very different smell. People who have never seen any Chinese medicine before may imagine that the herbs must be to do with Chinese cooking, and are the kind of herbs that are kept on a kitchen shelf. But, please, do not expect to be able to use them in a salad dressing!

Chinese herbal medicine consists of herbs, flowers, seeds, fruit, bark, root, etc. Although most of the medicines are derived from various plants, a small percentage are also made up of a motley array of minerals, shellfish, and some animal products.

The taste of these medicines vary; most have a very strong flavour. Although we occasionally do use a single herb, in most cases, we use a "prescription" which is a mixture of between 10 and 15 dried herbs. So, the taste is a bit like a mixture of coffee, sugar, pepper, salt and vinegar! Although some patients actually like the taste, there are a few people who cannot face drinking it. But Chinese herbal medicines should not be mixed with food unless the patient is a baby, whose taste buds have not developed fully.

What do Chinese herbal medicines contain?

The chemical compositions of Chinese herbal medicines are very complicated. Every herb contains many different ingredients; in most cases, the effectiveness of a herb is from its particular combination of ingredients.

The most common compositions in Chinese herbal medicine are as follows:

Alkaloids

Alkaloids containing nitrogen can be found in many medicinal plants. Alkaloids are one of the most important active ingredients in Chinese medicine. There are many different types of alkaloids which exist within different plants: some are effective for treating cancer, some relieve pain, some are good for asthma, etc. The alkaloids cannot usually be dissolved in water directly; most of them exist in plants as a form of salt combined with organic acid. Therefore, by cooking the herbs in water, we can extract many of the ingredients in the plant.

Cardiac glycosides

Cardiac glycosides are usually found in seeds, bark, and plant roots. They consist of a combination of a sugar with a non-sugar, the latter of which is the more physiologically active. There are also many different types of cardiac glycosides: some can act as diuretics, some can strengthen the heart muscles, some can cause diarrhoea, so can be used to treat constipation, and many of them have antibacterial effects.

Tannin

As the name suggests, tannin is used to tan leather. It gives the Chinese herbal concoction a very strong, dark reddish-brown colour. That is why when the herbal liquid spills on clothes, it is quite difficult to wash off. Tannin exists mostly in seeds, bark, root and leaf, but there are hardly any in flowers.

It has a very strong astringent taste, similar to the taste of pomegranate skins or even orange peel. Depending on the astringency, tannin can help to cure coughing, bleeding, diarrhoea and infections.

Volatile oils

These are oils taken from plants. They are not very stable and can easily evaporate when heated. Almost all aromatic herbs (such as peppermint, ginger, angelica root, peony root, rose, etc.) contain volatile oil. Strong-smelling herbs are normally good for the digestion: for moving the vital energy to expel the external "wind". Colds, flu and aches and pains in the meridians are caused by "wind".

Organic acids

Organic acid is more concentrated in unripe fruits. The best known organic acid is Vitamin C or ascorbic acid. Other organic acids are citric, tartaric and salicylic acids. Some of these acids are anti-bacterial or mildly diuretic. In Chinese medicine, the acid taste is supposed to be good for the liver, since liver and sour taste both belong to wood in the Five Elements theory.

Resin

Resin can also be an active ingredient in Chinese medicine. It can act as an antiseptic, helps stop bleeding, relieve pain and is used as a pesticide.

Others

Other, less important, ingredients include starch, tree gum, protein, sugar, colouring, fibre, etc. These ingredients may not directly participate in the healing process, but can reduce the side effects of the active ingredients.

Is Chinese herbal medicine safe?

Strictly speaking, no medicine is completely safe, not even herbal medicine. Unless it is used properly any medicine could cause problems. For example, the famous Chinese herb *Ginseng*, is a tonic herb that is famous for its energy-giving properties. Because of this, people mistakenly think they can take it as often as they like. But too much *Ginseng*, or the wrong type, can cause headaches, nose bleeds or insomnia.

Chinese medical theory holds that illness is somehow related to the imbalance of Yin and Yang, so treatment involves rebalancing them. All herbs have different Yin or Yang properties, so, if somebody is suffering from fatigue caused by a deficiency of Yin, then herbs that have a Yin property, or cold nature, should be used and vice versa.

There are several different types of *Ginseng*: *White Ginseng*, *Red Ginseng*, *American Ginseng*, *Korean Ginseng*, etc. Although they are all used as tonic herbs, their effectiveness can be quite different. Their properties can be extremely hot or extremely cold. Therefore, if you don't know what is the cause of your tiredness, you may risk making the Yin-Yang in your body even more unbalanced by taking the wrong *Ginseng*. Then there is the dosage: the normal dose for an adult should be around 3–6g per day. Patients have been known to die from an overdose of *Ginseng*.

The effectiveness of herbs used in Chinese medicine is well documented. Open any TCM pharmacopoeia and you will find not only the effectiveness of the herbs described but also the possible side effects; which herbs are relatively safe, and which herbs are not; which herbs can be mixed together and which can't; as well as recommended daily dosages. Although most of the herbs are very safe each one has its limited dose. A properly trained practitioner would not prescribe any herb over its limited dose range.

What are the different types of Ginseng?

Chinese Ginseng (Paeonies ginseng) is regarded as "the king of tonic herbs" and is one of the most popular tonic herbs used in China. Basically, there are two different types of *Ginseng*: the *White Ginseng* and the *Red Ginseng*. The *White Ginseng* is raw and its colour is cream or slightly yellow. Once it is cooked (usually steamed to prevent the loss of the effective ingredient), its colour turns to a reddish-brown and it is called *Red Ginseng*.

The nature of the most common *White Ginseng* is neutral, with a slightly bitter-sweet taste. It can be used as a general tonic herb for fatigue and feeling weak. Since its nature is neither too cold nor too hot, it can be used to treat both a Yin- or Yang-deficient condition. It can also improve appetite and help insomnia.

The *American Ginseng* (paeonies quinquefolium) is a different species from the Chinese one, but is also classed as *White Ginseng*, since its effectiveness is similar to that of Chinese *White Ginseng*, although its nature is cooler than the Chinese one. Apart from having the effectiveness of a general tonic, it can also be used to tonify the Yin, and cool the body system to treat a hot condition such as a dry mouth with sore throat and constipation.

Red Ginseng (cooked *Ginseng*) or the *Korean Ginseng* have relatively warm natures so are good for cold symptoms, or Yang-deficient conditions, such as an aversion to cold, bad blood circulation or even diarrhoea in the early morning. *Red Ginseng* can also be used for other Yang-deficient conditions caused by weakness such as breathlessness, dizziness, blurred vision, etc. Very heavy periods with light red blood are caused by a deficiency of Yang-*qi*. *Red Ginseng* can also be used in emergencies to stop bleeding and shock.

How much should I take?

For those who have never taken any *Ginseng* before, starting with 3g a day is a sensible dose, since a large dose of *Ginseng* can cause insomnia (if the person becomes too energetic!), nose bleeding or even nausea. If taking *Ginseng* powder or tablets, the dose should be smaller, approximately half of the dose of the raw *Ginseng* root.

In an emergency, when too much bleeding causes cold sweats, cold limbs and low blood pressure, it may be worth trying either *White* or *Red Ginseng*. Take a 9–15g *Ginseng* capsule with water or use 15–30g *Ginseng* root, soak for half an hour, simmer for 40 minutes, and get the patient to drink the liquid immediately.

How should I cook Ginseng? And when should I take it?

Ginseng should be steamed rather than boiled, since very high temperatures may destroy its active ingredient. First, soak the *Ginseng* with 150ml of cold water in a mug for one hour or overnight in the fridge, then sit the mug in a saucepan with some water in and the lid on, bring it to the boil, then simmer for 40 minutes. When it cools down, drink the liquid and eat the root if you wish. It is better to take *Ginseng* in the morning before food, because then you absorb more. If necessary, take it twice a day, once in the morning and once in the evening before food.

Should I avoid some food while I take Ginseng?

Turnips and tea should be avoided since they may reduce the effectiveness of *Ginseng*.

According to modern research *Ginseng* strengthens the heart and raises the blood pressure, so a patient with very high blood pressure should not take a big dose of *Ginseng*.

People suffering from a cold or flu or a high fever caused by infection, should not take *Ginseng*. *Ginseng* is for treating weak conditions, not excessive conditions.

Are there many different forms of Chinese herbal medicine?

Yes. There are pills, powders, plaster, paste, ointment and dry loose herbs. The most popular form is loose herbs, since they can be freshly made up for every individual person.

Loose herbs are usually prescribed for acute or serious cases, but for chronic and less serious cases, pill forms are often used. Sometimes patients can start with loose herbs and when their condition improves, they can change to the pill form to continue the gentle healing process.

Skin conditions are often treated with ointments, creams or lotions alongside the herbal "tea". The external medicine can work directly on the skin lesion, while the internal medicine balances the Yin and Yang, and eliminates the cause.

What should I expect to be asked when I go to see the TCM practitioner?

Normally, almost anything that you think is related to your illness, even if it doesn't seem to be relevant, is important to the practitioner. A good TCM practitioner will always pick up any information that might help them to make more accurate diagnoses. TCM practitioners make diagnoses individually, according to different patients. For instance, you may go to see a practitioner for your eczema. You may have been told that the cause of your eczema is an allergy, and prescribed a steroid cream. But, according to the Chinese medical theory, one of the causes of eczema is a weak spleen, so loose stools, bloated tummy and poor appetite, are all signs to look out for. So, when you go to see a TCM doctor, your tongue and pulse will be checked and you should expect to be asked about your bowel movements, your period cycle, your sleep pattern, whether you feel more thirsty than normal, whether you prefer hot or cold drinks, whether you perspire a lot, or have night sweats, etc. This is all very important information that can help the practitioner to determine their diagnosis for your particular case.

How much does it cost?

Most TCM practitioners in Britain would expect you to pay between £20 and £35 for the initial consultation. Subsequent consultations are cheaper. Loose herbal mixtures normally cost no more than £2–£4 per day, depending on your age and condition; acute conditions need a larger dose and shorter treatment than chronic conditions.

Can Chinese medicine cure eczema?

The Chinese for eczema is *Shi Zheng*, which means "wet rash", because most Chinese eczema sufferers have weeping lesions, and most of them can be cured. Only a very few patients' eczema becomes chronic. Unfortunately, most eczema sufferers in Britain suffer from "dry" eczema, which we call atopic dermatitis. This is usually a chronic condition, and apart from different steroid creams and antihistamine tablets, little can be done to relieve the symptoms.

However, the effect of Chinese herbs on eczema was discovered a few years ago almost by chance by Dr David Atherton, a consultant dermatologist who worked at both St. Thomas's Hospital and the Hospital for Sick Children in Great Ormond Street. At the time, the dermatological department of St Thomas's was in a small street in London's Chinatown; in this same street there is a female Chinese doctor, Dr Luo, from Canton in southern China who treats her patients in a tiny herbal shop using traditional Chinese herbal medicine.

A few of Dr Atherton's patients also went to see Dr Luo and the results surprised Dr Atherton, since many of these patients had been using different steroids for years with little effect. However, after taking Dr Luo's herbal remedies, their skin condition improved. As a result, Dr Atherton referred many more patients to Dr Luo, most of whose conditions also improved markedly. With the evidence mounting, Dr Atherton decided to visit this Chinese doctor.

So, for the first time, a conventional doctor in the West had started to communicate with a doctor from the Far East in her herbal shop. Naturally, their discussions centred on the treatment of eczema, the most common skin complaint in this country. The Chinese doctor agreed to give Dr Atherton a few herbal medicine formulae for eczema so that he could begin some clinical research on it, although she was adamant that, according to traditional Chinese medical theory, each patient must have a different treatment with an individual prescription.

As Dr Atherton later wrote in his book *Eczema in Childhood: The Facts* (Oxford University Press): "The possible therapeutic effectiveness of this type of treatment was first brought to my own attention several years ago, when a boy under my care with severe atopic eczema was taken to see a Chinese doctor in London's Chinatown area. He was treated with a daily decoction prepared from a mixture of dried herbs. This treatment proved impressively successful for him, and there were no obvious adverse effects.

"Subsequently, more than 30 other children under my care were treated in this way by the same Chinese doctor, and we observed a sustained and marked improvement in about 75 per cent of them. In many cases, the eczema was severe and had not been adequately controlled by any of the full range of currently available orthodox treatments in the UK.

"We felt we were now in a position to undertake a full-scale clinical trial of one of these formulas, ... At the end of the study, ... We regard a 60 per cent improvement in a child's scores as indicating a very worthwhile benefit from treatment, and it was calculated an improvement at least as good as this was observed in the majority of the children . . . . "

In 1992, Dr Atherton and his colleagues published their research article in *The Lancet*. As a direct result of this story, in April 1993, BBC television made a documentary about Dr Luo, her cure, and Dr Atherton's research team at Great Ormond Street Hospital; it was broadcast on the popular *QED* programme. As well as making us feel more sympathetic to the eczema patients and their families, it also made us wonder whether we should turn our backs on traditional medicine? Although western medicine has invented wonderful things like painkillers, there was nothing to combat the itchiness of eczema; the only palliatives were steroids and antihistamines, which were not only of little use but also had unwanted long-term side effects. The only thing patients could do to comfort themselves was scratch until they bled.

What other conditions can Chinese medicine treat?

Chinese herbs are particularly good for treating ("wet") eczema, psoriasis, headaches, menstrual problems, PMT, chronic fatigue, aches and pains and digestive problems.

How long does it take for the herbs to start working?

Many people think that because herbs are much gentler than western medicines, they will take relatively longer to work. In fact, herbal medicine can work very quickly; most prescriptions involving decoction rather than pills can start to work within a few days. But, whatever form of Chinese herbal medicine you are going to take, you should see some signs of improvement within a few days, or a few weeks, depending on the length and the severity of your illness. If you do not respond to one remedy quickly enough, an amended prescription will be given. So the gap between the first and the second consultation should not be too long.

How long should the treatment last?

Depending on the condition, it can last from a few days to a few months, sometimes up to two years. It really depends on the illness. If it is an acute condition, such as a cold or flu, a cough, diarrhoea or stomach ache caused by food poisoning, several days of treatment would be enough. For a chronic condition, like eczema, psoriasis, migraine, arthritis, ME or irritable bowel syndrome, it would take longer.

With herbal treatment, should my condition get worse before it gets better?

No. If, after taking the herbs, the condition gets worse, don't panic, just contact your practitioner as soon as possible. Only very rarely does a patient have an allergic reaction to the herbs. In some cases it could be as a result of stopping the medicine you were previously taking. Many patients might think the herbs can work miracles, but if the previous medicine you were using is much stronger than the herb, its effect on your body system will stay for quite a long time. For instance, if you have been using a steroid cream for a long time, and you stop it suddenly, your skin condition will get worse. So, if you stopped using the steroid cream just before starting to take herbs, you may mistakenly think your skin condition was caused by the herbs. Sometimes it can confuse the practitioner. So, you must consult your doctor before abandoning a course of treatment as well as informing your herbal practitioner of any medication you have been taking.

Are there any side effects of herbal medicine?

The most common reaction, or side effect as you might like to call it, from taking the herbs, is that of loose bowels. The patient may have more wind, and the bowels move more frequently. The cool nature of some herbs can make the bowel movements more frequent, even cause diarrhoea, so if you are suffering from irritable bowel syndrome, you must tell your practitioner so s/he can use a different formula to improve that while treating your other disorder.

What is the difference between Chinese herbal medicine and European herbal medicine?

Just as Chinese herbal medicine can be traced back thousands of years so European herbal medicine can also be traced back to the first people who lived in Europe. Although western herbal medicine is not as popular as conventional medicine, there are still quite a few herbal medical schools in Europe, to train practitioners.

The main difference is that each Chinese herb can be used not only for one or two symptoms, such as headache and fever, throat infection and cold, but for many other conditions, depending on what other herbs are being used. The interaction of the herbs is taken into account and several herbs are prescribed at once rather than just a single herb.

Are there any animal products in Chinese herbal medicine?

Chinese medicine contains not only herbs, but also minerals, some animal products, and other plants like bark and seeds from bushes or trees. Since most Chinese medicines are derived from plants, vegetarians can receive treatment. Practitioners will use alternative herbs instead of animal products if you prefer. There are a lot of substitute herbs that can be used just as effectively as the animal products, but you must tell the practitioner before the start of the treatment.

Does Chinese medicine use any products derived from endangered species?

For thousands of years, people believed that tiger bone could cure rheumatism, because the strong tiger bone would be able to strengthen the weak damaged human bone. The tiger, like the other endangered species (panda and elephant), are now protected animals in China, and the penalty for killing these animals is death. Therefore, a properly trained practitioner would not use tiger products. Practitioners on the Register of Chinese Herbal Medicine do not use any products from endangered species.

Preparing the herbs

Do the herbs have to be soaked before being cooked? Yes; all the herbs we use are dry herbs, not fresh ones. Most of the herbs will have been sliced or chopped into small pieces for easy cooking, but there are still some that are dry and thick, which take a long time to be totally soaked. If the herbs are cooked without soaking, or not soaked for long enough, the water can't get into the centre of the herbs, so many of the ingredients will not dissolve into the decoction, even after cooking. Herbs must be soaked in cold water before cooking, to ensure that they are soaked right through since if the herbs are roots, hot water may soak the outer layer of the root well, leaving the inside of the root dry and hard.

How long should herbs be soaked for?

Usually about 30 minutes for leaves, flowers, or other soft materials. Seeds, roots and minerals should be soaked for 60 minutes. If you have to leave them overnight they must be kept in the fridge. If the herbs are dusty, or not clean enough, you can wash them first, then soak them in cold water. After soaking, use the same water to cook the herbs.

How much water should I use to soak the herbs?

This depends on the amount and type of the herbs. For instance, leaves and flowers are lighter than minerals and roots; the former absorb more water than the latter. There are several ways of measuring the water; here are the two commonest ones:

1) *The traditional way*
Put the herbs in a saucepan, evenly covering the bottom. Cover the herbs with 2–3cm (1 inch) of cold water. This is the easiest, but least accurate, method of measuring the water.

2) *Using a measure*
For most herbs, for the first cooking add 500–700ml (about 1 pint) water. For the second cooking, use relatively less water: 300–400ml (about 1/2–3/4 pint).

Cooking tonic herbs takes longer so they need more water. For the first cooking use 700–900ml (about 1 1/2 pints) water; for the second cooking use 400–450ml (about 3/4 pint) water.

Herbs for colds or flu are normally light and contain more volatile oil, so need less cooking time. For the first cooking, use about 400–600ml (3/4 pint to 1 pint) water and for the second one use 250–300ml (1/2 pint) water.

How should I regulate the temperature?

This is very important. There are two types of heat: slow and fast. With fast heat the temperature rises very quickly and the water evaporates very fast. Pungent herbs for treating colds and flu must be cooked with fast heat to keep the main ingredients from evaporating. Some herbs for constipation should also be cooked with fast heat in case they lose their effectiveness. But most tonic herbs must be cooked with slow heat to let the ingredients dissolve in the water as much as possible. In most cases, we start with fast heat and continue with slow heat, stirring every 10 minutes.

How long should I cook the herbs for?

Again, it depends on the herbs; normally they should be cooked for 30 minutes after boiling for the first cooking, and for 20 minutes after boiling for the second cooking, but the pungent herbs that usually contain a lot of volatile oil (these are usually in the form of leaves or flowers) don't need much cooking: the first cooking for 10–15 minutes, and the second cooking for 5–10 minutes. Most tonic herbs are in root form and take longer to cook: the first cooking should last about 60 minutes and the second cooking about 30 minutes.

What if I burn the herbs?

If the herbs are burnt, the active ingredients are destroyed, so their effectiveness would be diminished.

Can any saucepan or pot be used to cook herbs?

In China, we use earthenware pots to cook herbs in because they transform heat evenly and slowly and are more stable than some metal ones. Aluminium saucepans can cause a chemical reaction with some herbal medicine and reduce the effectiveness of the herbs. So avoid aluminium, iron, copper or stainless steel pans. Enamel, glass and ceramic pans are good alternatives.

Can I cook herbs in the microwave?

It is not recommended, because it is difficult to control the temperature and the time in the microwave. The herbs might be cooked in a few minutes, but most of the active ingredients will still be in the herbs and will not have devolved into the decoction, so as we are not supposed to eat the herbs, a lot of the ingredients will be wasted.

Taking herbal medicine

Can babies have herbal treatment?

At the beginning of this century, China's first paediatrician, Qian Yi, developed many effective remedies for children's illnesses that are still used in modern China.

According to traditional Chinese medical theory, the kidneys are the foundation of the constitution, but the spleen (digestive system) is the source of nutrients for growth and development. As a baby's spleen is very delicate, many foods and medicines can weaken it, and this affects the baby's general constitution. In TCM, the spleen is supposed to be the most sensitive organ to herbs with a cold or bitter nature, so when we prescribe herbal medicine for a baby, we should be very careful not to use too many cold or bitter herbs. Babies should be given herbal medicine, when it is warm. As babies are very sensitive to medicine, their condition can be changed dramatically by a small dose of herbs over a very short period, so the practitioner should see baby patients frequently to monitor their condition.

How can you make babies take herbal tea?

Many Chinese herbal medicines have a bitter taste, but these can be avoided when treating babies. Herbs like orange peel, bamboo leaves and liquorice can have quite a nice taste, and most babies would drink them without too much trouble. If we start them on a very small dose they will slowly get used to the taste. If a bitter herb has to be used in the prescription, here are a few tips to make babies drink the "herbal tea".

With a smaller quantity of more concentrated medicine use a syringe to squirt the medicine to the back of the baby's throat, preventing the tongue from touching the medicine. This is only suitable for an older baby, since it requires their cooperation.

Hold the baby's nose so he cannot smell it.

Let him suck an ice cube to numb the tastebuds before giving him the medicine. Here are some other tricks:

Mix some fruit juice, milk or honey with the medicine to reduce the bitter taste. (Blackcurrant juice mixed with herbal tea tastes best.)

Taken cold, from the fridge, herbal tea tastes better than when it is warm.

Give the baby some grapes immediately after the herbal medicine.

Brushing the baby's teeth with a minty toothpaste before giving the medicine can reduce the taste.

How big a dose should a baby be given?

If the baby is still being breast fed, we might let the mother take the medicine so that the baby gets the treatment through the mother's milk.

As a general rule, for babies under one month, we recommend $1/6$ of adult dose; for babies under one year, $1/3$ of adult dose; for children under seven years, $2/3$ of adult dose; and for 7 to 12-year-olds, almost the same as an adult.

It does, of course, depend on the type of herbal medicine; on how many different herbs in a prescription, on the strength of the herbs used, etc.

Should pregnant women take herbal tea?

If you are pregnant, before you start to take herbal medicine, you must tell your practitioner. Although most herbal medicines are quite safe for pregnant women, there are some that could be dangerous. For example, some herbs for arthritis intended to "move" the blood and help the circulation, may also cause miscarriage. Most tonic herbs are perfectly safe to be taken during pregnancy, but others, such as diuretic herbs, herbs for constipation, cancer or psoriasis, are quite harsh and care is needed. Special care is needed in the early stages of pregnancy (6–11 weeks). But that doesn't mean avoid any treatment; if the mother is not healthy, how can she have a healthy baby?

Can sugar be used with the "tea" to mask the unpleasant taste?

This is not a good idea. The effectiveness of Chinese herbal medicine is determined by taste: most tonic herbs have a sweet taste (liquorice/dates) whereas herbs used to clear heat, etc. have a bitter taste, so if we add sweet sugar to bitter tea, the taste would be a bit better, but the effectiveness might be less strong as well.

On the other hand, most sweet foods increase heat in the body, and if we want to use the herbs to clear the heat, but add sugar to them, we may "add fuel to the fire". So, it is better not to add sugar unless your practitioner agrees.

What food should I avoid while taking herbal medicine?

In Chinese this is called *Ji Kou* (food taboo).

In China medicine and food are very difficult to tell apart as some medicines are used as food and some foods are used as medicines. "Food and medicine come from the same source" is a famous saying. A medicine's effectiveness is determined by its different taste and nature: sweet, salty or pungent taste and hot or cold, the same goes for food. A patient who suffers from a cold condition, such as diarrhoea, shouldn't eat cold or raw food; a patient who suffers from a chronic cough and has a deficiency of Yin shouldn't eat too much spicy or pungent food.

Can I take herbal medicine with other medication?

Most herbal medicines are natural products, like food. Most of the herbs can be used with other drugs without any side effects. In China, herbal medicine is often used in conjunction with modern western medicine to treat complicated cases. Both medicines used together often produce better results. For instance, chemotherapy or radiotherapy are two major cancer treatments in modern medicine and, as we all know, this kind of treatment can be very toxic, because the drugs or the radio-therapy will not only kill the cancer cells but also lots of normal healthy cells or tissue as well. According to TCM theory, patients who suffer from cancer have very weak *qi* (vital energy) so some very strong herbs are needed to treat it, which we explain as "using poisonous drugs to expel the evil factors", but at the same time, we use tonic herbs to strengthen the *qi* and build up the immune system. Herbal medicine can also relieve side effects, such as sickness, poor appetite, etc.

But some herbal medicines may reduce the effectiveness of certain antibiotics.

If I feel sick after taking the herbs what should I do?

The bitter taste and strong smell of the medicine can make patients feel sick after taking it. There are a few ways to relieve the nausea:

1) *Ginger*
Press about 50g of fresh ginger to extract the juice, mix it with the herbal tea and drink it. Ginger is used in Chinese medicine as an anti-emetic and is good for colds.

2) *Wet flannel*
Soak a wet flannel in hot water, wring it out, and while it is still warm, compress it around the neck, then drink the tea.

Other ways of relieving nausea include making the tea more concentrated and drinking less, drinking it warm, drinking it slowly, not all in one go.

Should herbal tea be drunk cold or hot?

In most cases, drink it warm although generally speaking, for hot conditions drink it cold and for cold conditions, drink it warm.

When should I drink the tea (before or after food)?

Tonic herbs should be drunk before food; and diuretic herbs are better drunk on an empty stomach. Very bitter, pungent or sour herbal tea should be drunk after food. Herbal tea for insomnia should be drunk before going to bed.

Should I drink the sediment?

Although some of the ingredients from the herbs can be dissolved in water, there are still many that can't be dissolved in water, such as starch and some minerals. These sink to the bottom and should be drunk otherwise you may miss some important ingredients.

Tonic and health

When is the best season to take the tonic herbs?

Basically, we can use tonic herbs at any time. But traditionally, in China, we take tonic herbs mostly in the winter because winter is the time to restore energy and keep healthy. All the plants are very quiet until spring when everything in nature starts to wake up, and in summer, with the help of the sunshine, everything grows very fast, and autumn is the time to harvest.

So we still have this custom of taking more tonic herbs in the winter. *Dong Zhi* is the date in the Chinese calendar that indicates the start of winter. So this is a good time to buy tonic herbs or food for your parents or grandparents, to wish them a long and healthy life.

What kind of tonic herbs are suitable for me?

The best thing to do is consult a herbalist. There are a few common tonic herbs or food such as *Ginseng*, for general weakness (there are several different kinds of *Ginseng*, see page 131, and different people should take different ones according to their condition), and white or black wood ear (the white one is for tonifying the lungs, Yin for people who suffer from chronic bronchitis or asthma; the black one is for tonifying the blood and kidneys).

The red or black dates are also very common for tonifying the blood and *qi*. Sesame seeds and walnuts are good for the blood and kidney Yang. Cinnamon is also good for kidney Yang.

Which is better for tonification: food or medicine?

In China it is said that tonifying with medicine is not as good as tonifying with food. Most people believe that minor ailments can be nursed back to health by eating proper food. If the illness is more severe, then we should take herbal medicine, because it is stronger. However, if it is not used properly, herbal medicine can do more harm than good, so it is always advisable to consult a specialist before taking any tonic herbal medicine.

10
The future of Traditional Chinese Medicine

The future of Traditional Chinese Medicine has always been unpredictable. Once it even went into crisis when the Guo Ming Dang Government nearly banned it because it was "not scientific".

It is a healing art, based on ancient philosophy and rich clinical experience.

Traditional medicine should develop in its own way, just as it has done for centuries. Science has obviously influenced traditional medicine in some ways and will always do so. For instance, acupuncture is the result of developments in the metallurgical industry. Before the acupuncture needle was made, people used acupressure instead of acupuncture. Medical books dating back 2,000 years show that the acupuncture meridians and points were already there, but some form of sharp stones were used instead of acupuncture needles.

Modern western medicine can learn much from traditional medicine, but modern medicine should not be used to interpret traditional medicine, otherwise traditional medicine will eventually lose its own spirit and value, and be replaced by modern medicine. For instance, herbal medicine cannot be tested on guinea pigs because guinea pigs are different from human beings, and one of the main principles of TCM is that a proper diagnosis has to be based on the individual.

As a healing art, the future of Traditional Chinese Medicine is unpredictable. Whether it will be developed or lost in the next century depends on the support of patients, the government, and most importantly, the practitioners.

Useful addresses

The Chrysanthemum Clinic
3 Station Parade
Burlington Lane
Chiswick
London W4 3HD
TEL: 0181 995 1355

The Register of Chinese Herbal Medicine
9 Lawns Court
The Avenue
Wembley Park
Middlesex HA9 9PN
TEL: 0181 908 1697

The School of Chinese Medicine
Principal: Michael McIntyre
Midsummer Cottage
Nether Westcote
Kingham
Oxfordshire OX7 6SD
TEL: 01993 830419

Further reading

1. Atherton, David J., *Eczema in Childhood: The Facts* (Oxford University Press).
2. Compiled and translated by Bensky, Dan and Andrew Gamble, *Chinese Herbal Medicine: Materia Medica* (Eastland Press).
3. Compiled and translated by Bensky, Dan and Randall, *Chinese Herbal Medicine: Formulas and Strategies* (Eastland Press).
4. Kaptchuk, Ted, *Chinese Medicine: The Web that has no Weaver* (Rider).
5. Maciocia, Giovanni, *The Foundations of Chinese Medicine* (Churchill Livingstone).
6. Veith, Ilza, *The Yellow Emperor's Classic of Internal Medicine* (University of California Press).

Index

Page numbers in *italic* refer to the illustrations